Upside Down
to Rightside Up
Daily Inspirations for Fitness

Jade Krauss Thornton

WALDENHOUSE PUBLISHERS, INC.
WALDEN, TENNESSEE

Upside Down to Right Side Up: Daily Inspirations for Fitness

Cover art by Barbara J. Smith
QR codes and illustrations by Chan Williams
Edited by Jennifer Dickerman, Kelly Ferguson, Kelly McSwain, Scott Logan, Patsy Harris, and Charles Smith
Type and Design by Karen Paul Stone
Published by Waldenhouse Publishers, Inc.
100 Clegg Street, Signal Mountain, Tennessee 37377 USA
423-886-2721 www.waldenhouse.com
Printed in the United States of America
ISBN: 978-1-947589-69-8
Library of Congress Control Number: 2023930287

Upside Down To Right Side Up offers daily fitness inspirations and YouTube videos for every day of the year. This book gives tips on the right mindset, confidence, and motivation to make health and wellness part of everyone's daily walk. Fitness is for everyone! You can do fitness! -- provided by Publisher.

DISCLAIMER: Not all exercise is suitable for everyone. As with any exercise program, if at any point during your workout you begin to feel faint, dizzy, or have physical discomfort, you should stop immediately. Please be advised that by participating in any of the exercises presented herein, you are assuming all risks of injury that might result. You are responsible for exercising within your limits and seeking medical advise and attention as appropriate. The owner, its parents, subsidiaries, affiliates, participants of this book and videos, *You Can Do Fitness*, shall not be liable for any claims for injuries or damages resulting from use of the content in this book and any related videos. We further disclaim any liability caused by intentional or unintentional negligence. The information presented herein is not a substitute for medical advice. To reduce the risk of injury, consult your doctor before beginning this or any exercise program.

HEA007000 HEALTH & FITNESS / Exercise / General
HEA007050 HEALTH & FITNESS / Exercise / Strength Training
SEL027000 SELF-HELP / Personal Growth / Success

Dedication

I dedicate this book to the two souls who changed my life forever: my daughters, Zephany and Zadrian.

As soon as I saw the whites of your eyes from birth, I raised the bar of living to a standard of Godliness and excellence. I wanted the very best for my girls. During the years of raising you, you both gave me the courage to start my own business and go for the visions and dreams God placed in me long, long ago. I love you, Zephany and Zadrian, more than words could ever describe! I wouldn't take back the years we had as "a three pack" for anything. I am extremely proud of the two self-sufficient hard-working adults that you've become.

Last but surely not least! My husband, Bob.

You're the love of my life. The good Lord blessed me far beyond my every expectation. If it weren't for you, none of this would be possible! I love you with every fiber of my being!

Contents

Editor Recognition

I want to thank every editor who has been involved in this writing process. When I first got the vision from the Lord in 2008, one of my dearest friends, Patsy Harris, not only helped me articulate my heart on paper and edit my articles, she helped me get *You Can Do Fitness, LLC* off the ground from payment structure to seminars to personal support. She was a lifeline in helping me get through those first brutal years when I lost everything I stood for as I learned about the devastating unknown acts of my first husband. She helped with trying to fumble my children in the court system, finding a job to support my children, a place to live, and a car to drive. So much more she did for me … I'm forever grateful to her.

Next came Scott Logan, who was also a great demonstrator of God's love in helping me with my articles (beyond placing punctuation in proper places). He was my English teacher and taught me so much more than what an editor is supposed to do.

Then along came my mom's husband, Charles Smith. He is a renowned retired educator in the school systems. I can't thank him enough!

My sister, Kelly McSwain, has been a huge part of my life. She has also helped me articulate what I'm trying to convey in this book. Her support has been supernatural, and if I wrote about all the things she's done for me it would take an entire book itself. I value not only our sisterhood, but our sisterhood in Christ.

Toward the end of this editing process, I met a lovely, lovely lady and fellow author, Kelly Ferguson. She is so long-suffering, gracious, and understanding. I can't thank her enough for helping me articulate beyond just a simple period or explanation point. Due to unforeseen circumstances, she had to step down, but her help will never ever be forgotten.

In completion, the Lord brought to mind a sweet lady I had the honor to begin a fitness coaching relationship with during Covid. I didn't realize she was exactly what I needed. She took on this project as if it was her own. To name a few things, her dedication, excellence, precision, and brilliance have blessed me beyond measure. She's the type of person everyone wants to be around. She gets things accomplished. I'm extremely thankful for Jennifer Dickerman's help in finalizing this project.

I can't thank you guys enough for working with me. As you all know, I have major learning disabilities and needed your help far beyond what an editor is supposed to do. I love you guys and I'm forever grateful for your help!

Prologue

When I say my passion is fitness, I mean it has truly been my lifelong "friend" that has helped me cope with all the ups and downs of my life. Ever since I can remember, one of my most prominent characteristics has been my strength. I was never a good student due to learning disabilities, but I could arm wrestle the football team, and I could throw the cheerleaders up in the air (just like the guys do now, but this was before there were guys on a squad). We all gravitate toward our strengths to be accepted by others, so I buried myself in exercise to cover my learning challenges. Not being very smart drew me down a road of extreme insecurity and self-destruction until I turned thirty years old.

My dad had been praying for me for years. He often called me when I lived in Florida and asked numerous times for me to move back home. I had just won a fitness title and walked off stage with offers from national competitions in New York and Hollywood, California, but strangely, it was then that I agreed to move back to Knoxville, TN with my dad. Looking back, I truly believe that it was the power of prayer from others that gave me this out-of-character desire to turn down these other offers and move home.

Choosing a new life direction and moving in with my dad at thirty years old was, needless to say, difficult and awkward. My dad was a great help in it all, but he had a couple of rules. He offered for me to live with him short term while I attended Massage Therapy School and worked in the local gyms to get on my feet. His biggest rule was I had to go to church with him every Sunday while under his roof.

I think it was the first Sunday that I was back at home when my life changed forever. I felt a nudge as the last song was playing at my dad's church, and the pastor made an altar call. I really and truly thought that my dad and the pastor had talked, and the altar was waiting for me. So, I grabbed my dad's hand, and we went up front together. My sister and I had gone out the night before, so I was still in party mode, and I had no idea what was about to happen when we got up front. I bowed my head and said a prayer with a quaint group of people, which unbeknownst to me, were the people that had been interceding for my soul for years. Still half lit from the night before, I opened my eyes, and I did a 180° turn with my life right then and there. I went back to my sister in the audience and told her, "I feel so different."

This was my "Right Side Up" moment. Ever since that day, back in 1997, I have never been the same. I began to get acquainted with the Word Of God, and that was how I learned to live life right side up. From that moment on, I had a confidant, lover of my soul, provider, and protector. Jesus became my everything, and he was what I was looking for all along! I have been through things that some people never recover from and was often asked how I was still sane and standing. I'm here to tell you. I'm more sane than ever before and living life according to the Word of God. It's been one adventurous journey, and as I continue to fall down lots lately, I know where to run to, and Jesus ALWAYS picks me up and turns me right side up.

You may be wondering why I write about my story of fitness and faith and how it relates to you. I share my story with you because I know you have had some hard hits in life, too. None of us are exempt from hard things, so what gets you through? We all need something to believe in, in order to first believe in ourselves and help the people around us. I think I'm safe to say that all of us have some upside down stuff in our lives, and we come to a point of not knowing how to get right side up.

With a faith to hold onto and something constructive to do with ourselves, like fitness, we can overcome anything! I believe that we all have a specific calling to fulfill, and we can stay sharp in our life's purpose as we stay in shape to carry out the call. What do you say...? Let's all move forward with our faith and fitness and when the day gets you upside down, by golly, we know how to carry on right side up! Hold onto your faith and fitness and share your story to help others!

Jade Krauss
jadekrauss@gmail.com
You Can Do Fitness

FIRST QUARTER
Daily Inspirations for Fitness

Let's Get Started
Days 1-90

Scan the QR Code for each day
to take you to a companion
YouTube Video Workout

Happy New Year!
Day 1

The New Year is here. My hope and prayer for you is that you'll find a love for fitness. You will find your unique fit self and never be sedentary again. I have designed a special movement just for you to discover. My great hope is to set you in the direction of a lifetime of exuberant fitness.

Though there are guidelines to go by as you discover your personal plan, there are three training categories that we all need in our different quests. I'd like to share them so we can begin on the same page:

Cardiovascular training. If you're the type of person who has a tendency to be uptight and stressed, you may want your main focus to be on cardiovascular training, such as walking, biking, running, and swimming. As you focus on your particular cardiovascular routine, you are releasing stress chemicals by allowing more oxygen to reach your muscles, and you're tuning up cardiovascular endurance all at the same time.

Resistance training. If you're INTENSE, strength training is a great main focus. I personally am very intense, so I enjoy pushing and pulling some serious weight to start my workouts. Strength (resistance) training can be accomplished by you exercising with me.

Flexibility training. If you're the type of person who loathes that bubbly, off-the-wall instructor, or the gym scene, a quiet, group-led class or a home stretch/yoga video may be best for you. Stretching classes provide better functional abilities, such as reaching, bending, and stooping during daily tasks.

As you seek out your personalized fitness plan, feel free to contact me. We need ALL three categories. Choose a main category you shine in, but you mustn't forget the other two categories.

I'm excited to do fitness with you this year.

Insanity or Sanity?
Day 2

At the first of a new year, there's always a lot of anticipation with expectation. People want positive change to crisis situations and answers for better endings. In all the current chaos and hope for answers, it's a must to take daily care of ourselves, because like my daddy always told me, "There is a fine line between insanity and sanity."

We must do all we can to stay on the right side of the "sanity line," and physical exercise can help keep our mental health in check. The definition of mental health is: a state of well-being in which an individual realizes his or her own abilities, can cope with normal stresses of life, can work productively, and is able to make a contribution to his or her community. As we are waiting out the home stretch, let's care for our bodies and, in turn, our minds.

Listed below are a few ways exercise helps us mentally.

• Regular exercise can help improve mental health and mood, and extend lifespan. Exercise benefits everyone.

• Exercise helps brain health. Exercise pumps blood to the brain, which can help you think more clearly. It also stimulates the mind. It increases the connections between the nerve cells in the brain. This improves your memory and helps protect your brain against injury and disease.

• Regular exercise helps you get better sleep. Getting a high-quality, proper night's rest is another one of the benefits of exercise. Because regular exercise increases the physical temperature of your body, your brain can have an easier time winding down when you want to sleep at night.

As you move forward in life, proceed with MUCH hope. Don't neglect your mental health. I encourage you to push toward sanity and keep insanity at bay.

Mark ... Set ... Go!
Day 3

During this first week of the new year, you've determined goals to achieve. Goals always remind me of "The Tortoise and the Hare" story. There are "hare" people in life, goal oriented and quick to conquer, and "tortoise" people, slow and steady through and through. The perfect combo for success is slow and steady. The tortoise DID win the race.

Every single year, I have clients prove over and over again that "tortoises" win. I watch them take on just the right amount of exercise and nutrition, successfully meeting their goals. No one really wants to start in first gear. Doing a little bit of exercise and changing a few things in your eating is difficult. Working hard at a slow and steady pace takes more discipline, making it harder to stay the course.

The hare is a different story. Hare people start out with tremendous goals, sprinting right out of the gate totally determined. Soon the "hares" discover more breaks are necessary than expected. Hares end up frustrated and angry with themselves, asking the questions, "Why can't I do this?" "Why do I always find myself right back where I started?" "Why am I repeating the same old things I thought I had victory over?" We all want to jump right into fifth gear to get in shape quick. The truth is, there's no quick plan that lasts.

Being slow and steady gets a bad rap sometimes. The fastest "hares" seem to get all the praise. The wisest choices in life are made by going slow and steady. Maybe the hares can put a little intensity in the tortoise's life. Maybe the tortoises can put a little staying power in the hare's life. We need each other, especially the different personalities we bring to the table.

Here's his story: "I first thought about getting into fitness in July. It was then I started feeling a little self-conscious. I wasn't overweight or anything, but I wanted to make a change for me.

At 5'11", I was 185 pounds with a bigger belly than I was comfortable having. I finally found something I wanted to try, and it was the Insanity workout regimen. "Go big or go home," I suppose. This is a 9-week program. I added this workout in and didn't make any changes to my diet. I lost about 3 pounds. I repeated this workout regimen after a month break. This time I started watching my diet. I finished at 173 pounds, 12 pounds lighter.

I began tracking my body fat percent each month. I got my first measurement at 17.7% and 173 pounds. Starting with those numbers puts me at 30.6 pounds of body fat. If I remove the estimated 3 pounds of muscle and add the 15 pounds of body fat back to get to my weight of 185 before starting my fitness journey, I can reasonably assume that I started at 24.6% body fat.

My new focus was weightlifting. I lifted 2 days a week starting out. I was able to keep my muscle gain equal to my fat loss 5 months later. I still weighed 173 pounds but was at 11.8% body fat. This meant I was losing 2 pounds of body fat per month and also gaining 2 pounds of muscle per month. I wanted my muscle growth to outpace my fat loss by putting on more healthy weight and increased strength."

Client #1's testimony proves what ordinary days of lifting weights and eating right will do to produce extraordinary differences.

The Four-Step Process
Day 5

During our year together, I want you to be on the lookout for the four-step progression process. My videos are designed to get you moving. Then, as you progress in your fitness, you'll notice room for growth. Your consistency and faithfulness will bring results and physical improvements. My hope for you in the four-step process is that you'll be changed forever.

Let me share:

Step 1 - Get Moving! This step is designed for the beginning exerciser or the person who has not included a fitness activity in their life for quite some time. My videos will teach you the fundamentals of fitness and how little time it takes to make a difference. I'll bring you instruction, demonstration, and practical routines in each video.

Step 2 - Give Me More! You'll be noticing an improvement in your mobility and endurance levels. In addition to the encouragement for increasing your cardio workout, you can also add more resistance to each exercise in your daily video workouts.

Step 3 - Your Improvements Are Showing! Maybe your goal is to lose weight, or maybe it's just to walk through the mall without having to sit down 3 times. Your testimony will develop and have a positive impact on how your workouts have made a difference in your life. You'll continue to increase your exercise intensity without increasing your exercise time.

Step 4 - Welcome to Your New Life! Exercise will no longer feel like a forced activity, but instead it will be an exciting and welcomed part of your life.

My goal is to share my love for fitness (that will always benefit you). My prayer is your health will become a never-ending endeavor you pursue for a lifetime.

I challenge you to embrace this new year with high expectations for your optimal health.

Aspire ... Do It ... and Be All You Can Be

Day 6

rest day   You're on a hot trail for a better you. A lot of weight-loss testimonials saturate the TV. They're inspiring. I come from the fitness era (1980's) where you had very few role models. Men had Arnold Schwarzenegger and women had Jane Fonda.

Times have changed; now the industry is saturated with role models. You have an exorbitance of programs to get fit. In seeking your own unique way, find your personal zone.

Your personal zone helps you make the most of your workouts. This is found through the Karvonen Formula. This individual zone maximizes your heart work while increasing muscle and fat loss.

Here is the formula:

1. Take the number 220, then subtract your age.

2. Take that number and subtract your resting heart rate (your resting heart rate is most accurate when you count your pulse for 60 seconds first thing in the morning).

3. Take #2 and multiply it by 0.60 (this is your low zone).

4. Then take #2 again, but multiply it by 0.80 (this is your top zone).

5. This last step will give you your TARGET HEART RATE ZONE. Take #3 (low zone) and add back in your resting heart rate. Then take #4 (top zone) and add back in your resting heart rate. These particular numbers leave you with your personalized range.

After each workout, take a 10-second pulse and the number you count multiplied by 6 will reflect if you're exercising to your full potential. If you are exercising in your personal zone, then you can be confident that you are receiving the maximum benefit.

I hope you continue soaring to unbelievably new heights this New Year. Stay encouraged.

Geared to Win
Day 7

rest day

I'd like to help you get into a steady gear with your health and wellness. Let's begin in first gear until it's time for second, third, fourth, fifth, and then cruise control.

Let's break down these particular gears one at a time. Usually, everyone is wanting to get to cruise control in a week, including myself. Results take time. During this process, I want to set you up for a win-win.

1st gear: Start with a determination that whatever comes your way, you will eliminate the quit button.

2nd gear: Make up your mind NOW that your results will vary. Allow your body to mold and transform the way it's designed to be.

3rd gear: Once you have your mindset right, it's time to make time. When do you have the most energy? Will you be better committed to exercise in the morning or evening? You don't know? Try exercising when you enjoy exercising the most. It might be lunchtime or after work.

4th gear: When you've established your time frame, make sure you have a balanced workout regime of cardiovascular training plus resistance training. If you happen to need help with a balanced workout plan, you can contact me to help you.

5th gear: Diet is almost like a bad word. Everyone has a particular diet whether it is good or bad. Seek healthy dietary options.

Cruise control: You've found your fitness groove; you have your perfect balanced diet and fitness plan. Stay aware of when it's time to change things up to keep your body in response mode.

I encourage you to gear up toward the right direction for a win-win. Rise up and allow yourself to be who YOU are and celebrate how YOU are supposed to look.

Counting Blessings for a New Year
Day 8

I bet you have extremely HIGH hopes for your health this New Year. As you look to your future with the right perspective, it's a must to keep it simple and focus on what is really important. Taking time to count your blessings is always a great way to start the new year.

Faith: We all have faith in something. Faith is the substance of things hoped for and the evidence of things not seen. In simpler terms, there's something you've hoped for that has not yet manifested. Maybe you have faith for a better year, a better job, a better relationship with your spouse or a child, etc.

Health: Being thankful for the simple things like legs to move, hands to hold your loved ones, dumbbells, or straight bars; a functioning body, living disease free, and overall good health. Let's not sweat the small stuff or get bent out of shape about not being the "perfect number" on the scale.

Family: Now that another year is behind you, I'm sure at one time or another you've had concern over a loved one. Perspectives change as the years go by. A new appreciation for the simple things becomes most treasured.

Jobs: We must always consider the means to provide for our families. As we go forward into a whole new year employed or on a new adventure of finding employment, I'm sure we all agree that a job is something really big and should be counted as a blessing.

I encourage you to take on whatever the new year brings with the RIGHT perspective. CHEERS to faith, health, family, friends, and jobs. I challenge you to stay grounded in the simplicity of life and go forward in thanksgiving.

New Year Boost
Day 9

There's no better month than January to get a good handle on the New Year. Let's kickstart this year together by omitting our vices and begin eating and exercising the way we know we should.

We need a starting point, so I would like you to weigh yourself today and write down what it is. You can e-mail me your weight for the accountability, if that helps you. Set a goal to do my classes.

Now the eating and exercising begins. For the month of January, we will eat great and exercise on a consistent basis. Good food choices go a long way, and we will quickly see that truth revealed on the scale when we weigh in again at the end of the month. Any weight lost or weight maintained should be considered a success.

Sometimes we need a little push to jumpstart us, and what better time to start than NOW?! I'm excited that we'll be doing this together. I'll even be joining in on the fun by making some food sacrifices myself.

There's no better time than now time to make this commitment together. You are guaranteed to have no regrets. So what do you say? Let's get weighed in this week and kick-off a great year with a healthier you. Doing something new to better yourself is always a win. Change is inevitable; we might as well steer it toward staying the best we can be.

The Alternative

The first full week into this year is behind you. I'll bet you've already been tempted in some way to break your New Year's resolutions. It seems when you set your mind to doing well and taking action...BOOM! You stare temptation in the face. Don't do it. Just think about the alternative. If you don't decide to change, you will stay the same.

When all the hype is gone, it's about those old, familiar, and comfortable ways that creep back in. Be careful. Each small slip-up can pave the way for you to continue making similar mistakes in succession. This pattern is known as behavioral momentum. Your behavioral momentum is like a snowball effect. You can let behavioral momentum drag you down, or you can use it to push you toward any healthy goal.

At first glance, a New Year's resolution to lose weight, eat better, or exercise more can seem daunting and overwhelming. However, by breaking down your goal and using behavioral momentum, you can make steady progress through the weeks and months ahead.

I encourage you to take this approach. Watch out for extreme highs and lows while staying the course (this is hard for me because I'm so extreme in my thinking). I encourage you to make subtle choices. Rest assured, when you just do it, you will not only feel accomplished and encouraged, but you will also see results and reap rewards as well.

Come on. Take the road less traveled. The alternative is staying the same. Yuck! Stay the course. Your reward is waiting.

You Can Handle Challenges
Day 11

 Embrace "that one thing" that you've poked, prodded, and talked about but have actually never really done anything about.

Together, I'd like to embrace the challenge to make a change. Change is hard, but if we stay where we are, we simply keep circling the mountain. I want to climb the mountain of change this year. Commit to exercising with me this whole year.

Here are some ways to keep your commitment in the face of unforeseen challenges:

The starting point begins today. Begin with small goals like exercising with me, then add more goals when you're ready for more.

Set aside your exercise time. A new habit takes at least 3 weeks to become firmly established. It will take at least that much of a time commitment for most people to adapt the HABIT of exercising.

Movement. Move your body for at least ten minutes most days (four days or more). When you're ready for more, increase the duration, up the intensity, or try another type of exercise.

Work your muscles. You can work your muscles with me. See you on video!

Nutrition. Yep, welcome to my downfall. For most people interested in seeing results and losing body fat, this is by far the hardest, most important component to manipulate. By reducing your intake by 250 calories a day through exercise, you can lose a pound or two a week.

Let's discover the benefits of better health and wellness together. There is great freedom found in movement, using your muscles, and eating sensibly. Don't underestimate the power of fitness. I encourage you to take on this new year determined to not be the same. Be determined to be a stronger, more confident you. Your journey begins today.

Why Breakfast?
Day 12

The first month into becoming the new you, your routine still isn't where you'd like it to be. I have a suggestion - eat your breakfast. Did you know that breakfast stands for "break the fast?" When you eat breakfast, you are literally breaking a fast. You've fasted all night long. Now it's time to rise and shine and break your fast. This is a great way to begin your day, encouraged and strong.

Some people think that if they skip breakfast it will help them lose weight, but this common practice is more likely to cause weight gain than weight loss. Skipping meals, especially breakfast, can make weight control more difficult. Breakfast skippers tend to eat more food than usual at the next meal, or nibble on high-calorie snacks to stave off hunger.

Here are a couple of good, healthy options that will help you begin your day on the right foot:

An omelet. An egg-white omelet is an excellent protein-packed meal to start your day. Depending on your individual preference, you can add your favorite vegetables and seasoning to your omelet. You could add ground black pepper, cayenne pepper, crushed red peppers, fresh herbs, or hot sauce. The biggest thing to remember is to keep it interesting.

Oats and berries (if you're not an egg person). Rolled oats or steel cut oats are another great option. Oats are loaded with beneficial carbohydrates to give your muscles energy. Oatmeal also has a notable amount of fiber to keep your digestive tract functioning properly and to keep you feeling full. Berries add sweetness and more fiber.

If these two options don't really tickle your fancy, I encourage you to go on your own quest to find your perfect balance. Eating breakfast is a great routine.

Home Scale Types
Day 13

Do you have a home scale somewhere in your home? They are usually found in the same place in all home types, the closet or bathroom. A scale is a very primitive way in measuring someone's health and wellness in comparison to what is actually the truth about human body weight. A scale is so primitive that they will one day end up in museums.

Providers now offer the consumer way more than simply measuring body weight alone. When looking to purchase a home scale, it's a must to consider a scale that can measure more than just your weight (the mass number) - BMI, bone density, body fat percentage, etc.

For instance, you can purchase a Body Fat scale, which can measure both your body weight and estimated fat percentage. Or my friend told me that hers even tells you the BMI. The only downside of relying on the BMI charts for health goals is that it doesn't measure body fat. So, an athlete with a lot of muscle could have a higher BMI, which is solely based on height and weight.

If you are looking for a home scale, I would recommend you choose a scale with several measurement options, not just the total mass scale number. On the flipside, I wouldn't get too fancy, because too many ways of measuring could leave you confused and frustrated.

If you already own a standard scale, I wouldn't put too much clout in what it says. We must be reminded that scale weight is only a small part of health and wellness victory. Keep your eyes on the good things that are happening, not a silly number on the scale.

Happy Feet
Day 14

I'm sure you've heard the saying, "If momma ain't happy, ain't nobody happy." Well, this can also apply to your feet. If your feet ain't happy, ain't no workout happy.

How do you know if your feet are happy? Here are some things to consider.

It's important to buy a sports or training-specific shoe. For instance, if you're a runner, you need a running shoe. If you play baseball, you need a baseball shoe. If you're a Cross-fitter or a weightlifter you need a cross trainer shoe. Specific shoes provide the stability and support to meet specific training needs.

You must not let the outside of the shoe be your guide. When it's time for you to purchase a new pair of shoes, they will probably still look brand new. The treads of your running shoes or the looks of your training shoes could look like you've barely worn them. A good rule of thumb to go by for when it's time to replace them is how they feel.

What's the harm if you continue wearing worn-out shoes? Injuries. Worn out shoes are common causes of running injuries. It's been proven that worn out shoes increase the stress and impact on your legs and joints, which can lead to over use and chronic injuries.

Shoe insoles can provide support. Insoles are meant to be inserted into shoes to provide some relief from general aches and pain.

Unhappy feet can affect our whole body, especially our ankles, knees, hips, and lower back. New shoes really do go a long way. Remember, our feet need attention, too!! Back pain or annoying chronic shin splints just might go away with a new pair of shoes.

Are your feet happy today? I sure hope so.

Stretches For The Hip Flexors
Day 15

 Today, I'd like to share some specific stretches you can do for each particular hip flexor.

Did you know that the hip joint is one of our most flexible joints and allows a greater range of motion than all other joints in the body except for the shoulder?

Here are some specific stretches.

1. *Iliopsoas* stretch. Flatten the small of your back while lying flat and contract your abdominal muscles. Bring your knee to your chest while your other leg and the small of your back are touching the floor.

2. *Rectus Femoris* stretch. Lie on your back with both knees bent. Pull your left knee toward your chest as far as you can. Let right foot drop off the edge of the bed toward the floor.

3. *Sartorious* stretch. Kneel with one knee on the ground, the other bent at a 90-degree angle in front of you. Keep your spine upright and think of your pelvis as a bucket full of water. Lean forward with your spine still completely upright. Clenching your buttock muscles while you do this may help you get a feel for the right motion.

4. *Tensor fasciae latae* stretch. Standing position – cross your right leg behind your left leg. Your right foot should be to the outside of your left foot. With both feet pointing forward, lean the weight of your body over your right foot. Keep your hips pressing forward. Allow your left hip to drop slightly until you feel a stretch in your outer right hip.

5. Inner thigh muscles stretch. Toe touch – put both your feet together at the heels and slowly push on the knees with your elbows.

Let us continue to seek knowledge to better understand how to care for ourselves.

Sleep it Off
Day 16

One of the first things we do in the morning is to evaluate how we slept. If we are dragging, we may even evaluate how well we've slept all week. Sleep is extremely important. We've all experienced a lack of sleep from time to time and it's no fun. People who experience insomnia know what being severely exhausted feels like firsthand. It can be miserable.

Regular exercise can improve your quality of sleep. Regular exercise helps people fall asleep faster, spend more time in deep sleep, and awaken less often during the night. When we sleep, our bodies recover from the stresses of the day, rebuild damaged tissue, and restore health and energy reserves.

The good news is sleep is one of the most underrated tools of weight loss. However, on the other end of the spectrum, sleep deprivation can cause weight gain. Research presented at the 2006 American Thoracic Society International Conference showed women who slept five hours per night were more likely to experience major weight gain as compared to those who slept seven hours a night.

In addition to weight gain, a lack of sleep can also result in memory impairment, increased levels of frustration, reduced productivity, depressed immune system, and impaired judgment. Needless to say, these are not the qualities of life we work so hard to achieve by exercising.

As you plan your day, I encourage you to include enough movement to suffice for a quality night's sleep. Maybe set a goal to walk 10,000 steps. Don't forget to also plan your evening so that you get an adequate amount of sleep. Sounds like an odd thing to do, but you will find it is well worth your while.

Chronic and Acute Pain
Day 17

My brother and I were on the phone the other day, and he was complaining about pain in his knees. He recently started a new job that requires a lot of physical activity. The element of pain will always be with us and must be managed. My brother and I discussed what to do when new, mild pain occurs.

Let's clarify what mild pain is. Symptoms of mild pain usually consist of a sudden onset of pain, soreness, limited range of movement, bruising, swelling, or stiffness. In my brother's case, his knees were swollen and sore to the touch. An acute injury or mild pain occurs when your muscle is overstretched. This usually occurs as a result of fatigue, overuse, or improper use of a muscle. These common problems are known as a muscle strain, or muscle pull.

Strains can happen in any muscle, but they're most common in your lower back, neck, shoulder, and hamstring. All pain must immediately be assessed. If it's a severe muscle strain, it's typically a muscle that is severely torn and needs medical attention. My brother's injury was minor. I encouraged him on Friday to rest the whole weekend and apply the following principle:

The R.I.C.E. method

- Rest
- Ice
- Compression
- Elevation

By Sunday, my brother was 90% recovered. The moral to my little brother's story is the R.I.C.E. method works. This method only works with minor injuries that don't need medical attention. Going to the doctor is ALWAYS the safest bet. More severe strains may take months to heal and can turn into a chronic injury that needs medical care.

I encourage you to stay in the race of health and wellness by playing it safe.

Belly Fat
Day 18

If you had a choice of where you gained extra weight, I'm sure it wouldn't be in your belly. But, unfortunately, that is where it all goes. Some people struggle to lose belly fat more than others due to genetics. Whether you're genetically prone to belly fat or not, too much belly weight can be dangerous.

Getting rid of belly fat is important for more than just vanity's sake. Why is belly fat so dangerous? Excess abdominal fat, particularly visceral fat, is the fat that is stored within the abdominal cavity. It surrounds your organs, puffs your stomach, and may appear as a "beer gut."

This excess fat is what increases risk for heart disease, type 2 diabetes, insulin resistance, and some cancers. If diet and exercise haven't helped reduce your mid-section, then hormones, age, and other genetic factors may be the reason why. As you get older, your body changes how it gains and loses weight.

We can fight this process. The number one culprit is calorie consumption. You may be eating a healthy diet, but not be aware of how many calories you're consuming. One good way to know is to track your calories.

Aerobics help reduce excessive belly fat. Aerobic exercise is so effective because it elevates your heart rate to burn calories and see results. Doing hours of sit-ups won't help you reduce visceral fat like aerobic activity.

Strength training reduces belly fat, too. It helps tone, condition, and build muscles. When you build muscle, you increase your metabolism so that even at rest your body will burn more calories.

I wish I had a pill for getting rid of belly fat; I would share it! The truth of the matter is that the formula for reducing belly fat takes continual work and dedication.

Body Composition
Day 19

Over the years, my "scale number" has haunted me. It doesn't matter if it is a high number or low number, it's a bad trigger. If it's a high number, I get depressed and eat. If it's a low number, I want to celebrate and eat. I've always felt lost because I don't know what I should weigh.

Body composition is a great way to measure true weight. Body composition is the proportion of fat, muscle, and bone of an individual's body. There are three ways to measure body composition.

The most accurate measurement of body composition is (underwater) hydrostatic weight. This is a procedure for measuring underwater weight and is used to determine the body density versus fat percentage.

Bioelectrical impedance. Bioelectrical impedance measures the resistance of body tissues to the flow of a small, harmless electrical signal. As it sends this electrical current through the body it can determine body composition. Because lean mass contains more water, it takes the electrical current less time to travel through the body and assess composition. This type of measurement is typically assessed through hand-held devices or scales.

Skin folds. Skin fold calipers measure body fat by pinching visceral fat at specific anatomic locations, and those numbers are used in a formula to estimate total body-fat percentage. These are less accurate due to it being a challenge to measure at the exact anatomical site every time.

The next time you step on that scale, please take note that the "scale number" you're looking at is the weight of the gravitational pull on the body. It's your mass plus gravity. Do NOT get hung up on a number.

Aging Joints
Day 20

rest
day
When we age, lots of changes occur. If you're younger than 40, this fact is hard to believe because most people feel so good. When I was in my 20's and 30's, I didn't have much patience for older people standing around talking about body pain. Years later, the joke's on me. I have much more compassion for injuries and body pain.

I'd like to talk about the body's joints. The definition of a joint in human anatomy is the physical point of connection between two bones. All human joints contain a variety of fibrous connective tissue. Ligaments connect the bones to each other, tendons connect muscle to bone, and cartilage covers the ends of bones, providing cushioning.

I like to compare the ligaments, tendons, and cartilage (aka fibrous connective tissue) to a rubber band. A new rubber band is nice and smooth, somewhat like a 20/30 year old human joint. But after 40, our aging joints could be compared to an old rubber band.

Have you ever gotten a hold of an old rubber band that has disintegrated a bit? You can still use it but can't really trust that it will hold things together too well. After forty your joints simply need extra care. It's a must to find exercises that are easier on your less trusted joints. The stronger your muscles are, the less strain you're placing on your joints. You mustn't be afraid of weights.

Experiment with weight machines, free weights, and resistance bands: Start slowly and increase your intensity gradually. Experiment with cardiovascular machines, too. Spinning is a great option. The circular motion of cycling minimizes the jolting of traditional jogging.

Don't allow aging joints to keep you from utilizing some sort of fitness option. Have no fear, solutions can be found.

Body Fat Percentages
Day 21

rest day

When it comes to measuring your fitness success, the scale isn't always best. I had a client that had made tremendous strides in her fitness, but she hadn't lost a pound on the scale. She had gotten a lot stronger and diminished inches and body fat.

She said she's the type to only stay encouraged if she sees some sort of progress. I believe we all are like that. If we don't see some sort of progression, we're apt to quit.

There are other alternatives in charting your progress — one being body fat percentages.

Getting measured by a fitness professional is a great way to check your body fat percentages. Most people are afraid of fat and consider it an enemy that needs to be vigorously fought as it accumulates.

What exactly is an acceptable body fat percentage?

The Recommended Body Fat Percentile Range (Mayo Clinic)
Women:
20-40 yrs old: Underfat: under 21 percent, Healthy: 21-33 percent, Overweight: 33-39 percent, Obese: Over 39 percent
41-60 yrs old: Underfat: under 23 percent, Healthy: 23-35 percent, Overweight: 35-40 percent, Obese: over 40 percent
61-79 yrs old: Underfat: under 24 percent, Healthy: 24-36 percent, Overweight: 36-42 percent, Obese: over 42 percent
Men:
20-40 yrs old: Underfat: under 8 percent, Healthy: 8-19 percent, Overweight: 19-25 percent, Obese: over 25 percent
41-60 yrs old: Underfat: under 11 percent, Healthy: 11-22 percent, Overweight: 22-27 percent, Obese: over 27 percent
61-79 yrs old: Underfat: under 13 percent, Healthy: 13-25 percent, Overweight: 25-30 percent, Obese: over 30 percent

Caliper body fat measurements are a great way to chart your process and keep you encouraged. Make sure you don't get stuck on a number on the scale.

Change, Change, and More Change
Day 22

Whether we like it or not, our futures are headed for change. Truth be known, we won't make changes for the better until we experience some sort of pain. People make changes for good only when the pain of staying the same is greater than the pain of change.

Think about your point of view on the things in your life now and compare it to your point of view five years ago. I'll bet your views have changed. My wise pastor taught me during early years into adulthood: you have a sensational attitude to prove yourself in the world. In your mid-adult years, you have a drive to be successful at what you've chosen to do. As the years go by, you become sentimental looking back on life, realizing the things that really matter. Things simply change.

Your physical body will change. When we're young, we can't help but think we're indestructible. A decade ago I remember wanting to help this very attractive older lady thinking, "She's so pretty but her body would look so much better if she'd just tweak some things about her diet." How far from the truth that was. Learning for myself, 60-year-old thighs change and can no longer attain a 20-year-old's thighs, no matter how healthy you eat.

Change needs to be accepted and embraced. As you change, you can make it a goal to be the best you can be at your age. Place your focus on things that matter. Your physical body is not as important as how you treat others and what you do in this world to make it a better place.

We are only on this planet for a short time. I challenge you to look at each day as a gift.

Bladder Importance
Day 23

 If you are a parent, you understand the importance the doctor places on your newborn's bladder. If your infant's bladder is working properly, that's a sign of a healthy baby. If your baby gets sick, one of the first questions the nurse asks is, "When was the last time your baby had a wet diaper?" As we grow up, bladder issues are just as important, but it's not a very popular topic.

Let's see what's considered normal.

Have you ever wondered how many times a day you should empty your bladder? As with many things in life, everyone is different. For most people, normal frequency is about 6-7 times in a 24-hour period. These frequent visits play a big role in how much fluid you drink daily and the fluid types that you drink.

If you're taking any types of medication, they can affect your normal visits to the bathroom. For all of these reasons, it's good to make sure that you're staying well hydrated.

How do you know if you're hydrated? Doctors recommend to "Drink eight, 8-ounce glasses of water a day." Other signs of hydration are that you should rarely feel thirsty and your urine is colorless or light yellow.

There are some reasons you may want to see your doctor. Urinating too many times a day can indicate other serious problems, such as:

Diabetes

Prostate problems

Use of diuretics

Stroke

Overactive bladder

Urinary tract infection

The number of times a day you visit the restroom is a vital part of your health. Make sure you keep water accessible at all times for proper hydration. If you're thirsty, that's an indicator that you're too late and that you are dehydrated.

The moral to this story is your bladder does matter! Because YOU matter!

Tips That Bring Lasting Results
Day 24

Every single year on January 1st, the local gyms are packed! Everyone is gung-ho, bound and determined to lose those extra holiday pounds. I love the energy in the gym that time of year. Everyone is talking about their new fitness and nutrition goals and going after them with a vengeance. It's an awesome atmosphere.

Then, by the second week of February, 80% of the New Year's resolution gym crowd drops off. Participation dwindles back down to that same ol' same ol' 1-2% total volume for the rest of the year.

All Year Round Tips:

Shop well. It is more important than ever as the year progresses to continue to stock your kitchen with healthy foods. Have healthy snacks handy. The more convenient they are, the more likely you are to eat them.

Scheduled workouts. Remember, even if you reached your weight goal last year, you still need to work out to maintain that weight. There is no destination with exercise or nutrition; your body is constantly changing, so you might as well enjoy the journey.

No thank you. Every time you're offered goodies or treats, say, "no, thank you." Most people probably aren't even aware of how many times they are offered extra food. Be aware next time, and instead of saying, "I'll try a bite," say "no, thank you."

Hydrate. On average, our bodies are made up of 60% water. Water is like drinking magic juice. If you get in the habit of drinking water, your body will have what it needs. Increasing your water intake can equal guaranteed weight loss.

We need encouragement and the reminders of simple tasks that bring lasting results. Let us carry on for the rest of the year and embrace lasting results.

Saddle Up!
Day 25

I'd like to share something about being single but apply it to fitness. I'm reading *Right People, Right Place, Right Plan* by Jentezen Franklin. He wrote, "You can approach your single years in one of three ways: you can be a griper, a grabber, or a gripper."

I've heard a lot of griping over the years and I'm not exempt. Griping can become a dangerous tool for quitting and giving up. Some griping examples: "Exercise isn't working. I don't see any difference. I've actually gained weight from exercise. Exercise hurts. I don't like to sweat. I'm fat, white, and ugly." Sure, it's easy to find something to gripe about, but you must believe if you're exercising regularly, good things are happening.

Or are you a grabber? For years, I've witnessed clients come into the gym because their friend saw major results with kickboxing (for example). My client then becomes eager to try kickboxing to get those same results, even though they hate kickboxing. Then, they inevitably quit because they are doing something they hate. We can NOT grab the first thing that we know about fitness, get turned off, and never return again. We've got to approach all fitness as a learning curve.

Instead, you must grip a specific routine. It's necessary to seek out different fitness options until you find that perfect exercise routine that does your body best for the particular season of life you're in. We've got one body and it's time to saddle up and take hold of your own reins.

I challenge you to saddle up. Don't be a griper or a grabber - be a gripper.

High Intensity All the Time
Day 26

If I told you that the intensity of your workouts produced the best results, you'd work out at high intensity every workout. Right? The problem is working out at this "high-intensity level" a lot more than you should will result in feeling spent, burned out, or even getting injured. As the case with most things, too much of a good thing isn't good.

There is a specific workout designed for high intensity called "High Intensity Interval Training" (HIIT). HIIT workout strategies alternate short periods of intense anaerobic exercise with less-intense recovery periods. Adding a couple high intensity workouts to your weekly routine does produce greater results.

One HIIT workout could be implemented when a new exerciser is ready for more intensity. For the moderate exerciser, one or two times per week would be great. Make sure your HIIT day is followed by a lower intensity day of steady cardio training, or an activity such as yoga or body-weight strength training.

For the advanced exerciser, HIIT workouts should be done NO more than 4 times per week. Doing more than four days of HIIT workouts per week could lead to over training, tissue breakdown, and body fatigue. Not listening to your body's cues to rest, you could create injury that limits your ability to do any exercise at all. In order to stay in the game of fitness, do not exceed the four per week maximum and recover adequately.

High intensity all the time is NOT where it's at! Even though HIIT has allowed us to "train smarter, not longer" by engaging in these more intense workouts, we must apply wisdom. Your body needs time to heal itself after this kind of training. No matter what fitness level, I challenge you to try a HIIT class. Fitness is endless learning; enjoy it.

Are Planks Better Than Crunches?
Day 27

I've been asked this question many times. People often hear planks are better than basic crunches, but that is not necessarily true. We need to incorporate both into our weekly fitness routine.

One exercise is never the answer to optimal fitness. Variety is key! Life is full of movement, so the intent of any exercise session or program should be designed to enhance our ability to literally move through life with greater ease.

A plank is an isometric exercise which is an exercise performed with no movement. It's zero movement but not necessarily less work performance. While preforming a plank, the muscles get less blood flow so the waste products accumulate more rapidly. The end result is to maximize burning in the muscle.

Planking is one of the most beneficial core conditioning exercises. Not only do they develop our core muscles nicely, they also work out our glutes and hamstrings. These muscles support proper posture and improve balance.

Crunches function to strengthen our core muscles. Abdominal muscles are part of our body's 29 core muscles which are located mostly in the back, abdomen, and pelvis. Crunches not only strengthen these core muscles, but they also protect and support our backs as well.

The benefit of crunches is we build our ab muscles safely and effectively. Planking, considered an advanced exercise, places unnecessary pressure on the lower back. Simple crunches, however, safely develop an internal corset to hold in the gut.

We need both for optimal health. We just have to make them challenging to get the best results. Here's to a strong, healthy abdominal wall. You can do fitness!

Be Ready for Rough Terrain
Day 28

| rest |
| day |

Hard days are coming. That's not bad news, it's just truth that must be grasped in order to keep on keeping on.

As we work out day in and day out, week in and week out, month in and month out, year in and year out, we'll experience highs and lows. I like to look at my lows as rough terrain. If we're not careful with our lows, we could perceive them improperly. When that appointed time arrives and rough terrain is upon you, it's time to hold on a little tighter. You must push forward a little stronger and learn all you can, because this too shall pass.

Rough terrain is like plateaus. Plateaus are seasons where you see no change, you feel no change, and you hear no change. Beware, the truth is, something IS happening. Change is happening whether you're seeing things transpire physically or not.

It's similar to the four seasons of weather. Each season is preparing for the next; your "plateau" is preparing you for what is next. It's very important how you view the plateau, because if you get discouraged and give up, your next season might not look so good.

When a workout plateau occurs, your body has adjusted to the demands of your workouts. Your results seem to come to a halt. The scale won't move. Even during a workout, when you're experiencing a plateau, you may start to feel unmotivated, bored, and you don't feel like going to the gym.

Here are ways to successfully overcome during a plateau: try something new, keep your mind fit, check your nutrition, or even call a friend.

Be ready for rough terrain. You WILL make it to the other side. You've got more results and joy to experience in your fitness.

Metabolic Training Works for Me
Day 29

Back in the 1980's, it was very unusual for women to be in a gym. Times sure have changed for women and working out. Today's market is saturated with many ways to get fit. If you're in the market for something that works, maybe you can try my favorite — metabolic training.

What is metabolic training? It's cardiovascular interval training. It's designed to challenge your body with bouts of harder work followed by important rest intervals. This type of training is misinterpreted for a "workout until you puke." It's reputation keeps people afraid of training this way.

I'd like to walk you through a sample routine.

First, you warm up for 30 seconds at an easy to moderate intensity based on your fitness level. For example, body-weight squats: Warm up those hips by challenging your range of motion while squatting. Then pause to stretch. For example, place both hands on the inside of your front leg in a deep lunge. Reach the outside hand toward the sky, creating the most distance from one hand to another. Repeat the warmup/ stretch about 3 times.

After your warmup/stretch segment, begin the actual metabolic workout. This segment takes about 10 minutes.

A sample workout

Squat jumps for a continued 30 seconds.

Lunge switch jumps for 30 seconds.

Rest for 30 seconds.

Repeat to equal a total of 10 minutes.

If you're not a jumper, a variation is to do the above workout with no jumping. As you perform each exercise for 30 seconds, it should be done at the highest intensity you can safely maintain.

The ultimate goal is to safely complete a large amount of work in a short amount of time, based on individual fitness levels. Metabolic training is a great boost to your overall fitness.

Short-Term Goals = Long-Term Success
Day 30

How do we truly achieve long-term health and wellness success? For any successful adventure, a plan must be put in place. Homes aren't built without blueprints. Parents don't go to work without a plan for childcare. We need a plan.

Our plan needs to consist of short-term goals. Some good examples of short-term aerobic fitness goals might include: 30 minutes of running on a treadmill, three days a week; Walking briskly 20 minutes, four days a week; Jumping rope 15 minutes, four times per week; or Riding an exercise bike for 30 minutes, three times per week. These particular short-term goals will improve cardiovascular health by increasing your heart rate and giving your lungs a workout.

It's also a must to have short-term strength training goals. A good example of a short-term strength goal might be 15 repetitions of exercises on various muscle groups for at least 30 minutes, two days per week. To create resistance, you could use an exercise band or weights. Don't forget to include regular, measurable increases in resistance or weight as part of your plan. These short-term goals for strength training promote endurance, improve muscle tone, and increase metabolism.

I challenge you to get your plan in place. Remember, short-term goals generally take four to six weeks to achieve. Think of short-term goals as stepping stones that are guaranteed to lead you to ultimate long-term success.

Get out your planner now and begin your individual plan today. God made you special. He wants to use you for the long haul. You need long-term success. You can do this.

Can I Benefit from Maxing Out?
Day 31

The biggest request all year round is weight loss. I constantly remind clients about strength, too. Both men and women need to gain strength. Today, I'd like to talk about maxing out.

"Why in the world would I want to max out?" a girl might ask. Maxing out with weights will take both men and women to new heights in their fitness level. It can even raise your metabolism, assisting the body to burn calories more effectively.

What is maxing out? Maxing out, aka Repetitive Maximum (RM), is performed through resistance training. This muscle strength is developed by the muscle contracting to its maximum potential at any given time. When you're going for the repetitive maximum on a bench press, you are stimulating your maximum voluntary contraction (MVC).

How can you personally meet resistance training goals by applying MVC? This is accomplished by manipulation of the number of repetitions (reps), sets, tempo, exercises, and force to overload a group of muscles and produce the desired change in strength, endurance, size, or shape.

Specific combinations of reps, sets, exercises, resistance, and force will determine the type of muscle development you achieve. General guidelines, using the RM range, include:

1. Muscle power: 1 to 6 RM per set, performed explosively
2. Muscle strength/power: 3 to 12 RM per set, fast or controlled
3. Muscle strength/size: 6 to 20 RM per set, controlled
4. Muscle endurance: 15 to 20 or more RM per set, controlled

Once you have sufficient experience in resistance training with support of a qualified fitness specialist or health professional, you might consider maxing out.

Your muscles respond in size and strength as they are forced to adapt. There are so many things to try with exercise. I encourage you to learn your body all you can.

The Extras of Winter
Day 32

Cold weather takes on a whole new meaning every winter. We all seem to forget just how cold the winter months can be. Due to freezing temperatures, your workout regimen needs some adjustments.

Cold weather can create a whole new set of exercise challenges. I like to call these challenges the "extras of winter." Whether you exercise all year round or have just started, winter time brings out the "extras" in us.

For example, you may feel extra tired, extra slow, extra stiff, extra irritable, and sometimes extra old. It would be easy to let any one of these items get in the way of your exercise plan. With fitness goals to achieve, you don't want these extras getting in your way of better health and wellness.

There is a key component for keeping you going this winter. The answer is increasing your warm-up time. By implementing this productive "winter extra," it will safeguard you against the "winter extras" that work against you. This "winter extra" will surely keep you in the game of fitness.

Adding extra warm-up time to your exercise routine provides more opportunity for your blood to get moving, your muscles and joints to get limber, your brain to become more alert, and your general body temperature to rise. Taking the extra time to warm up will do wonders in derailing the winter extras.

When you feel the "extras" coming on you, leave no room for negotiation. Get to the gym. Simply plan for a few extra warm-up minutes. You'll be glad you did! Winter will be over before you know it, and your perseverance during these cold days will be obvious come spring.

Winter Workout Recovery
Day 33

Have you discovered your body responding differently in cold weather? You're not crazy. The body does additional work to keep your body temperature regulated. As you train in the cold conditions, like a morning jog, your body is working extra hard. As you breathe, inhaling the cold, dry air causes your body to warm and humidify that air. With every exhale, you lose substantial amounts of water.

Although you may not have a desire to drink as much in the cold, replacing that lost water is essential so you don't become dehydrated. Dehydration is one of the main culprits for reduced performance and poor recovery in the cold. While it's harder on our body in the winter to respond simply because it's cold, make sure you emphasize drinking your water.

After a good winter workout a good recovery snack helps. Snacking properly will ensure you get the right kinds of nutrients, which will speed up recovery. Chocolate milk is a great recovery replenisher. When you are searching for the perfect chocolate milk, make sure you avoid pre-packaged chocolate mixes, which may contain artificial ingredients and excessive amounts of sugar. Instead, make your chocolate milk from scratch, with low-fat milk and melted dark chocolate.

Another great recovery snack is buckwheat pancakes. Buckwheat is a good source of protein, carbohydrates, and fiber. It's also naturally gluten-free. Instead of topping the pancakes with sugary maple syrup, you could replace the syrup with almonds and berries. You can even add honey, which possesses anti-inflammatory properties and the carbohydrates needed to help rebuild muscle fibers.

Be wise these next few months about what foods you use to recover from your workout and hydration, too. Work on your bikini/swimsuit body now. In April you'll have no regrets.

Guaranteed
Day 34

rest
day
If you're still exercising in the month of February, congratulations! You've officially reached a mile-marker. Did you know January 12th of every year is national quit day? On January 1st the gym is packed, but come January 12th, people have already thrown in the towel. IF you continue moving your body in some form of aerobic activity and make some effort to eat healthy, your results will be guaranteed.

It's true. All those gym equipment commercials that say "money back guaranteed if you don't get results" aren't lying. If you follow a plan and use your gym equipment, you WILL receive results.

Steps that guarantee results:

You MUST do cardiovascular training most days within a week. This means you need to move your body continually for 20 plus minutes at least 4 days a week.

One day a week of resistance training can make a BIG difference. That's anything that requires you to lift some sort of weight. This kind of training is so much more important than people think it is. Lifting weights makes your bones stronger, which allows you to live a longer, better quality life.

In Galatians 6:9 it says, "And let us not lose heart and grow weary and faint in acting nobly and doing right, for in due time and at the appointed season we shall reap, if we do not loosen and relax our courage and faint." That's so good in so many ways.

As it relates to fitness, do NOT grow weary in going to the gym and in eating what you know you should, because in due season, you'll wake up one ordinary morning and be gloriously surprised. Maybe you need to buy new clothes because you've lost weight or you feel fantastic with tons of energy. Your season is coming.

Facts About Hypertension
Day 35

rest day Hypertension is an abnormal blood pressure reading. The normal range for a blood pressure reading is the systolic (top number) should be less than 120, and the diastolic (lower number) should be less than 80. Therefore, 120/80 is considered a good healthy range. On the other hand, a hypertension type (high blood pressure) reading is systolic of 140 and greater, and a diastolic of 90 and over. So, 140/90 is considered a hypertension reading.

These readings are important because an abnormal reading can detect problems that can lead to serious health issues. As a matter of fact, untreated hypertension is a leading cause of heart attack, stroke, and kidney failure. It is critical to treat elevated blood pressure, since approximately 60 million Americans have hypertension.

Hypertension is often called "the silent killer" because a person may be unaware of elevated readings. 30 percent of the adult hypertensive population are unaware they have elevated blood pressure. All of the above facts signify the importance of regular blood pressure screenings.

See your doctor. Your doctor can prescribe medications that can help lower your blood pressure. Hypertension can be successfully treated with medications.

Hypertensive individuals who exercise regularly for several months can expect to see a 5 to 10 point reduction in both systolic and diastolic blood pressure readings.

It's best that individuals get their blood pressure checked on a regular basis to make sure their values are being kept within the desirable range. In many cases, individuals will need to be medicated to achieve desirable readings; even if blood pressure is not reduced with exercise training, the hypertensive individual should still exercise to help with weight management and for improvement of blood sugar control.

I encourage you to take all precautions to keep healthier living a priority! Because you matter!

Does it Really Matter What I Wear While I Exercise?
Day 36

Yes, it does matter what you wear while exercising. As a matter of fact, it's just as important as bringing water with you. Clothing has many functions, and it is important to choose the right outfit for the activity you are performing, as well as for the conditions in which you will be performing.

Here are some precautionary measures to take into consideration.

If you are exercising outside, you need to consider the weather. In cold weather, choosing easily layered clothing allows you to remove clothes as you heat up and add layers if you become chilled from sweat. A face mask or scarf is important, too. Its use is to protect your lungs from the cold air, and gloves and warm socks can protect your hands and feet.

In hot weather, the right clothing can help prevent heat-related illnesses. Loose clothing allows air to cool your body and evaporate sweat. Choose light colors instead of dark to reflect the sun's rays away from your body.

Wear the proper shoes. As shock absorbers, your feet are subjected to a lot of pressure during an hour of strenuous exercise. Proper footwear is important to cushion these loads. Different sports have different requirements for footwear, and it's beneficial to wear sports-specific shoes.

Water. You treat it like clothing. You can even buy a cute water backpack (Camelbak), but a simple water bottle will do. While exercising, you can lose between 6-12 ounces of fluid for every 20 minutes of activity. This is one big reason why you weigh yourself after a hard workout. You can weigh up to 5 pounds less after a workout. After your workout, replenish properly.

What you wear matters. I challenge you to make sure you've put thought into this simple task. Be prepared.

The Body Speaks
Day 37

You can NOT ignore body pain! At some point in your fitness journey, you'll have to be able to decipher exercise pain versus exercise soreness.

Exercise soreness is a normal experience from an exercise workout plan that can and will create what's called "DOMS," which stands for Delayed Onset Muscle Soreness. The reason this is "normal" is because in the process of exercise, you will be breaking down muscle and tendon tissue. At appropriate levels, the body responds by rebuilding that tissue to be stronger and more productive.

Exercise pain, on the other hand, is very different. Pain in one of your muscles or joints after a workout is usually an indicator of an injury. It usually lasts for more than 48 hours and is brought on by a specific movement rather than general soreness with all movements.

Here are several techniques to avoid injury:

Body consciousness. Being aware when your body displays fatigue or muscle failure. You can avoid potential injury by recognizing the warning signs of fatigue and muscle failure. Solution: take a break.

Body posture awareness. Your posture is your physical support system. Maintaining posture during the stress of exercise drastically reduces your risk of injury. Working out with good posture successfully fatigues your joints and muscles without compromising your stability in the process.

Exercise systematically. All this means is you need to exercise your muscles evenly and functionally. Evenly means that you don't want to train just biceps and chest. You need to train opposing muscle groups to create an even pull on the joint/muscle area.

Remember, do NOT ignore your pain. Avoiding pain with exercise is more in your control than you think. Take control of your health and your future. We've got one chance at this awesome gift called LIFE!!

A Client's Testimony #2
Day 38

 I believe nothing speaks louder and is more motivating than a success story. Dedication to living healthy is hard. Sharing the success of others will, without a doubt, inspire you in your own journey.

Here is Client #2's journey: "I started losing weight because I hated being in pictures. When I started, I weighed around 315 pounds and had a 42" waist. I started replacing my work lunch breaks with gym sessions.

In the beginning, I was too heavy to run on the treadmill. I would spend an hour on the elliptical with music playing, trying to keep up. I used this method to shed around 40 pounds. Then I started hitting the treadmill for an hour. The goal wasn't to run fast, just to keep running. By January, I had lost over 100 pounds, brought my waist down to 32", and was running 5 miles Monday through Friday.

I decided it was time to start lifting weights and try to bulk up in a muscular way. I dropped my Mon/Wed/Thurs runs to begin an upper body weight circuit. Tues/Thurs I was still doing my runs. It's unbelievable what happens to your body by adding weights.

My dieting techniques leave a lot to be desired. I'm an instant gratification type of person which I think is why I attempt crazy calorie counts and diets. If it weren't for keeping oatmeal cream pies around for my kids, my diet would be going a lot better."

My favorite part of Client #2's story is that he decided to make one simple change. He began replacing his lunch breaks with gym sessions. This small choice made extraordinary differences less than a year later!! AMAZING! Be encouraged! A healthy lifestyle ALWAYS equals a rewarding lifestyle.

You Burn More With Muscle
Day 39

There is one fact about health and wellness that will never change – muscle burns more calories. Yep, it's true. If you spend time lifting weights, whether that is going to a traditional gym, gardening, or housework to name a few, you're stimulating muscle and burning calories.

Muscle is a stimulus, and you are either placing your body in active environments that stimulate your muscles to grow (hypertrophy). Or you're placing your body in nonactive environments that don't stimulate your muscles so they shrink (atrophy). When you're constantly doing activities that build muscle, you are actually burning more calories simply to maintain your current muscle mass. Even on rest days, it takes more calories to maintain your muscle mass when strength training is a regular part of your weekly workouts.

So what do you do if you're not a gardener, hate house work, or are not too big on the gym scene? Below are a few suggestions:

- Push ups – on the floor or against the wall
- Squats – use a wall for balance if needed
- Lunges – either walking or in place
- Triceps – press back against wall or do dips using your furniture

(Note: Do this at your own risk and be careful that the furniture doesn't slip out from under you.)

People, when beginning their first fitness journey, often get confused about the difference between resistance training and cardiovascular training. Muscle is stimulated through resistance training: lifting, pushing, extending, and flexing. These are slow, controlled movements which are different activities from jogging and spin classes.

I challenge you to look at your week ahead and make a plan to either build more muscle or maintain the muscle you've developed. Choose specific activities that keep you challenged. Try keeping resistance routines on your weekly agenda. I guarantee you'll be amazed with your results!

Be Encouraged
Day 40

You can do anything you set your mind to. Sounds easy, doesn't it? However, the key is setting your mind to it. Fitness is no different; set your mind to achieving results. Accomplishing better health is possible. The stumbling block for most is that we set out with great intentions, only to find out that our body is willing but our mind is a bit reluctant. Our minds are working hard to convince us that we can't do this, that we can't make this change.

Be encouraged today that you can make this change. Allow your mind to accept the great things that you are doing for yourself. Not only are you making physical changes, but you're also making mental changes. Change in itself is hard. Stay alert and ready, knowing that with these changes comes challenges.

You can combat these challenges by asking yourself simple questions to stay on track and encouraged. Did you exercise one day last week? Be encouraged! Did you eat one less sweet treat at dinner? Be encouraged! Did you eat vegetables at one more meal? Be encouraged! Do you feel better than you have in a long time? Be encouraged!

Don't allow your mind to trick you into thinking that you are not working hard enough or that you need to do more to accomplish your fitness, health, and wellness goals.

I challenge you to allow your mind to let you celebrate your accomplishments. Encourage yourself in what you've set out to do, what you have been successful with, and what you've already achieved. Be encouraged. Keep looking forward and never give up.

Do Foam Rollers Really Work?
Day 41

rest day

I've personally experienced healing through massage therapy, and I've seen other people experience healing, too. The manipulation of soft tissue is so beneficial that I recommend everyone get massages regularly which can be costly. So if it's not in your budget, invest in a foam roller.

What does foam rolling do? It releases myofascia tissue like a massage does. These self-myofascial releases, also known as the "poor man's massage," can never completely replace a professional massage. They simply serve as great alternatives.

What are the benefits of using a foam roller? It increases blood flow throughout the body, allows better movement, and increases range of motion. It decreases the chance of injury and the recovery time needed after a workout.

How often can I use a foam roller? You can foam roll for 5 to 20 minutes each day, but even doing so a few times a week can make a big difference. Try rolling before or after workouts as often as you like. Foam rolling for 15-20 minutes and then stretching for 10-15 minutes before going to bed will help you sleep better, feel better, and recover faster.

I must warn you though. Foam rolling can be painful, even excruciatingly so, when you first start. Just stay with it for a few weeks, and the pain will ease up

Foam rolling is a great tool, but like no single exercise can give us optimal health, foam rolling cannot be the solution to all our muscle problems. It is always a good idea to see a doctor first for the proper advice on treating each particular problem. We'll better our chances for success by using our tools properly.

Benefits of Evening Exercise
Day 42

rest day

Exercising at any time of the day is beneficial, but there are some specific benefits of both evening and morning workouts. Today, I'd like to share some wonderful benefits of evening workouts.

Better muscle strength: there are differences in muscle performance between morning and evening exercise. When exercising at night, you have better muscle strength compared to exercising in the morning.

You may be able to stay at a higher intensity for a longer period than when you exercise in the morning. This may be important if you are doing any speed intervals for your exercise on certain days.

More energy: along with better muscle strength, exercising at night may give you more energy overall than during earlier times in the day.

Better sleep: a common reason for not exercising at night is that it may impair your ability to fall asleep. While this is true for some people, exercising at night may actually help some people fall asleep.

Releasing stress from your day: exercise is one of the healthiest ways to release stress. If you are stressed after a long day, exercising at night can be a great way to unwind. If you are prone to eat or just sit and watch television at night, try exercising instead.

The endorphins released from exercise can make you feel better and can put you in a better mood when you're done.

A frequently asked question is, "Do I exercise in the morning or evening for best results?" My answer is that it's ALL good. CHANGE that is done in an effective and safe manner is where the best results are found.

If you've never tried a morning workout, TRY IT. If you've never tried an evening workout, TRY IT. I challenge you to change things up.

Headache Relief Linked to Exercise
Day 43

Can working out relieve headaches? Absolutely! When you have a headache, the last thing you probably want to do is work out. Right? Sometimes working out is the best medicine for mild symptoms of sickness.

I would like to share how exercise can relieve a tension headache. A lack of adequate blood circulation is often the cause of a tension headache. Therefore, cardiovascular exercise is the best way to relieve a tension headache, because cardiovascular exercise helps with blood circulation.

This blood flow helps loosen and relieve tension in the muscles, which usually takes the headache away. The best types of cardiovascular exercises are walking, swimming, and cycling. Anything you can do to elevate your heart rate at a low intensity goes a long way.

Who would have ever thought? Exercising is like taking an aspirin. If there's no way you can even fathom moving your body, you can always stretch. Stretching loosens the tight muscles between your head and your neck.

Here are some exercises you can try to relieve a headache or even to prevent a headache:

Tuck your chin in toward your chest. Interlock your fingers behind your head. Gently press your head back into your hands. Hold this position for about 5 seconds and repeat this a few times.

Place your palms at the top of your forehead with your fingers facing back. Then move your palms in a rotating fashion making your skin move back and forth over your skull.

Grasp your earlobes, with your index fingers on the front part of the earlobes and your thumbs on the back of the earlobes. Gently pull your earlobes down and then outward in one smooth motion.

Consulting your physician is always top priority. There are many types of headaches. Exercise might be the medicine you need.

Sugar ... Need I Say No More?
Day 44

Yes, I said the word "Sugar," and yes, we're going there. I realize sugar is such a vast topic of discussion, but I'd like to skim the surface. I've been thinking about how exactly to approach a topic that I personally struggle with myself. A precious client of mine said, "Just give us the facts, Jade."

Sugar can be a part of a healthy diet if used in moderation. One of the first facts that's good to know is that 4 grams of sugar = 1 teaspoon. I encourage my clients to keep their daily sugar consumption to 10% (56 grams).

Our body metabolizes refined sugars at a supersonic rate. It's quickly broken down into glucose and fructose. The increase in glucose spikes insulin and blood sugar levels, giving you a quick surge of energy. If you do not use this energy immediately, your body may turn it into fat.

Fructose is metabolized in your liver and is absorbed at once, increasing fat cell production and workload on your liver. The quick digestion of refined sugar prevents fullness even after you eat a calorie-rich chocolate bar, leaving you hungry.

Before I close today, I must address fruit sugar. Fruit sugar contains many benefits compared to refined sugar. Fiber is found alongside fruit sugar. Fiber slows the overall digestion process, helping prevent increases in blood sugar and fat. Fruit, being fiber rich, makes its absorption different than that of refined sugars, which helps to improve your potty time and metabolism.

Refined sugars give you a spike in your metabolism and leave you sluggish and constipated, but don't be afraid of fruit sugar.

So there you have it – a few simple facts about sugar. I encourage you to go forward in moderation. #Hardestthingtodo

Safeguard Your Success
Day 45

How much are you willing to invest to protect your material possessions? We lock our doors and install security systems (even surveillance cameras) to protect the things money CAN buy. But what are we willing to do to protect our precious health (that money CAN'T buy)?

It's easy to become discontent in eating right, exercising, and lifting weights. We can all be like Scarlett O'Hara and say, "I haven't thought about that yet. I'll think about that tomorrow." The problem with Scarlett's thinking is those tomorrows can add up, and before long we've sabotaged our success. Let's be aware of the things that hinder us so subtly and easily.

One scenario: It's the weekend and some free time rolls around. You dart to the kitchen to make homemade cookies you've been craving all week long. You begin the process, only to find that when it's time to bake, you've eaten half the dough already. You cook the rest, still not satisfied. For some reason, we think calories don't count on the weekend, but they do.

Another scenario: You're out doing your weekly grocery shopping and huge party cupcakes find their way into your buggy. You get home thinking you better hurry up and eat four before the kids get home.

While these two scenarios might not resemble your life, I will confess they certainly have mine on occasion. I'll also confess that overindulgence is not worth the temporary pleasure it brings. The truth is, it leaves you with extra weight to deal with and depression that's hard to kick.

Let's stay away from the silent killers for assurance to safeguard our success. This frees you up to enjoy all facets of life. You'll be health-minded and ready to handle what life may bring you next.

Head Up, Shoulders Back
Day 46

Today's a great day for a pep talk. You will continue onward. You will keep your head high and shoulders back. You will continue in this race. If you've maintained your weight, applaud yourself. If you've gained weight, still applaud yourself. You're not going to quit. If you're experiencing victory, applaud yourself.

No matter what today holds, you will hold your head high and continue exercising. Even with only one month of this new year behind you, you've achieved some great mile markers by simply exercising. That alone should be commended.

When you implement exercise most days into your lifestyle, your body is more willing to extend a special grace for those days you mess up. For example, you've just returned from vacation and you've made some really bad decisions in the food department. You may be surprised that you haven't gained any weight. That's a benefit of regular exercise.

A rule of thumb is eighty percent of your success comes from what you eat. But, let's not underestimate the power of exercise to oppose your occasional food mess-ups.

When exercise is part of your DNA, your body recognizes food as fuel and is more apt to push the food through your body and use any "extra." Your body is simply more efficient, so when you exercise it's more likely to burn off the "extra" it's not used to.

Keep your head up and don't get one bit discouraged. You will keep up the great work. It's paying off. Not only will your body thank you for your choice to stay active, but when you fall down it won't hurt so badly.

Casein Protein
Day 47

What is casein protein? Casein protein is a milk protein. The major proteins in milk are casein and whey. These two milk proteins are both excellent sources of all the essential amino acids, but they differ in one important aspect. Whey is a fast-digesting protein and casein is a slow-digesting protein. Therefore, it's important to know the difference. This week we will take a good look at casein protein and next week we'll take a good look at whey protein.

Why would I need casein protein? Casein protein is the best food for your muscles, like milk is the best food for your baby's growth. If you're in the market for finding the perfect protein powder, all the different varieties may leave you feeling confused. With so many different options available to you, it can be a bit difficult trying to decide which is going to give you the best results and work in your favor to meet your specific goals. Casein may be just what you're looking for.

Here are some benefits of casein:

• Better muscle retention. Whenever you're going on a lower calorie diet, especially for men, there is going to be some loss of muscle mass. This is due to there not being enough calories to fully support all the energy needs required throughout the day.

• Higher quality protein. Casein protein is one of the best high quality sources of protein available. The body recognizes this source of protein as a healing property and keeps most muscle mass intact.

If you're into simple fitness, then a more basic protein powder will do. In the future we will discuss whey protein and its benefits. Casein may be a bit much for your liking. Learning will keep us in better health.

Contentment
Day 48

Success in health and wellness, as with most things in life, comes down to the basics. The basics of good nutrition, weightlifting, and cardiovascular training will never change. These basics have to be implemented for true lasting success, but there is an ongoing problem that is overlooked and often ignored.

This problem is people simply aren't content with being themselves. Contentment is the key factor that will bring sustainability. I like to look at contentment like a celebration. Celebrating yourself is a must in your health and wellness longevity.

I'm not encouraging arrogance. Rather, I'm encouraging you to be constantly aware of the small victories you've made along the way in your fitness journey. If you've lost weight … celebrate. If you shaved time off your run … celebrate. If you're eating healthy and feel better … celebrate. If you've kept a regular exercise regimen in the middle of the wheels coming off of your life … celebrate.

Once you've set your sails toward being content, we must add the proper commitments or it will erode our contentment.

Your goal should NOT be to lose 40 pounds in the next 12 weeks. Your goal should be to regain your health for the rest of your life.

Your goal should NOT be to bench press 300 pounds. Your goal should be to be the person who never misses a workout.

Your goal should NOT be to sacrifice everything to get your fastest time in next month's race. Your goal should be to be faster next year than you are today and faster two years from now than you will be next year.

I challenge you to set yourself up to win. Be content with who you are and committed to the end.

GOD does NOT make junk. You are a unique and beautiful person.

Sugar Alcohol
Day 49

rest day Have you ever read "sugar alcohol" on the "nutrition facts" of a food you're about to consume and wonder exactly what it is? Sugar Alcohol is a type of sweetener substitute. It's made from plant products such as fruits and berries. The carbohydrates in these plant products are altered through a chemical process to produce sugar alcohol.

Why would you want to eat sugar alcohol instead of real sugar? Sugar alcohol was made so you can consume foods that can pass through the body with minimal effect to your blood sugar and energy levels.

When you eat a candy bar, you get a big spike and then have a big drop in energy level due to the excessive amounts of sugar, unlike when you consume sugar alcohol. The body absorbs sugar alcohol differently and not as quickly as actual sugar.

There's also a difference in the number of calories. One gram of sugar contains four calories. One gram of sugar alcohol contains between 1.5 to 3 calories. This is one reason why sugar alcohols are found in a lot of diet foods.

Another reason foods contain sugar alcohols instead of sugar is so the food can be labeled as "sugar-free" or "no sugar added." If you're a Nutrition Facts label reader, then I'm sure you're aware that these sugar alcohols can be found in many foods such as chewing gum, sugar-free candies, cookies, and soft drinks.

Sugar alcohols may sound great by now; however, they do have some negatives. The most common side effects of consuming too much sugar alcohol include diarrhea and bloating.

I challenge you, just like everything else in life, to be moderate. Keeping food choices simple with a twist of moderation is always best.

Have Your Cake and Eat It, Too
Day 50

Let's do a daily protein intake check on ourselves. I'm going to help you. Did you know protein is essential for weight loss and body maintenance? In most cases, people are usually deficient in this area. For people who exercise on a regular basis, it is the one nutrient in particular that we need to be most aware of.

A quick trip into your body will reveal that it's constantly working to replace cells and tissue; it never gets a break. As regular exercisers, we are creating minuscule (tiny) tears in our muscles. Protein is essential in repairing those tears and making our muscles strong and efficient.

So how much protein do we need daily? As your personal trainer, I can safely prescribe that 15% of your daily caloric intake should be made up of lean proteins such as fish, chicken, tuna, lean beef, etc.

From my own personal experience, I've seen the value of including protein with each meal. I encourage you to do the same. Eating the foods your body requires first, such as your protein, is when you may indulge in an occasional fun food second.

Your body wants to work for you and not against you. Feed it the proteins, complex carbohydrates, fruits, and fats in the quantities it requires. Make sure you make the time to exercise because it craves movement.

Then, when you give your body what it's designed for, you'll find that it will shape up and respond beautifully. Following this lifestyle will allow you to not only look at the cake, but have a little once in a while, too.

Life's too short to not enjoy fun foods from time to time. Stay protein conscious and see what happens. Your body will thank you.

One Guarantee ... Things WILL Change!
Day 51

Things in life are guaranteed to change. Isn't that the truth? How about the 2020 pandemic? The uncertainty of the pandemic coming upon us so quickly has left us wondering about the future and all its unknowns.

I'd bet if I asked you if you've been stressed about something this past week, your answer would be, "Yes, I've experienced stress." I've got wonderful news in the midst of all the chaos in the world today. EXERCISE HELPS ELIMINATE STRESS.

I'm so thankful to be in this industry for this very reason. Through exercise, I can help people release stress. As stressful things are constantly coming your way, you must set aside extra time to move your body. One of the wonderful things about social media is it gives you access to people in the fitness industry. They're only a click away and willing to help you.

Don't allow yourself to go stir crazy living life with no healthy outlet. It's so important to stay mentally positive in these uncertain times. Negativity will only get you down, but by golly, we will hold our heads high, be constructive, and press forward. Nothing ever stays the same; whatever you're facing, this too shall pass.

During the interim of any stressful season, I challenge you to strive to use exercise as a constructive tool to eliminate unwanted stress. Then, no doubt, you'll come out on top.

I encourage you to be determined to make the best of every single part of your life. Always remember, if anyone needs help and guidance on how to implement your personal health and wellness, I'm just a click away. Exercise with me. See you on video in cyber space.

Being Too Full Isn't Cool
Day 52

Sometimes our food experiences trigger good memories that we love to relive. For instance, remember that cozy feeling you got as a child? It's raining, your favorite movies are on, and your mom was in the kitchen making your favorite cookies, popcorn, or meal? Or maybe in your first year of college you discovered a newfound freedom in eating and drinking.

Maybe it was when you met the love of your life and you found it to be so much fun eating together. These are all great memories! No one is wrong in longing to recreate their memories, but sometimes to eat now as we did then can leave us sedentary, sluggish, and even depressed: in most cases fighting unwanted pounds.

As bodies constantly change, what we previously enjoyed might not be as much fun for us anymore. Let's look to create some new experiences with how we exercise and eat. To do so, we may need to study up on the latest and greatest exercise moves that are appropriate and beneficial for each of us and on the exciting healthy food options available. Eating healthy doesn't have to be boring.

If research isn't your thing, then surround yourself with people who exercise and eat right. I know they would be excited to share their secrets with you.

Chasing old food memories may leave you feeling sluggish, sedentary, and stuffed full of unwanted food. It's easy to find ourselves seeking comfort found in the familiarity but end up in an endless pit.

The good news is, you can become a student in the school of health and wellness. It's the best school to attend: discovering trial and error, learning what works and what doesn't, and graduating from being too full of food, to embarking on new experiences and memories.

What About Alcohol?
Day 53

 I'm frequently asked the question, "What about alcohol?" Today, I think we should talk about it.

How does our body digest alcohol? Alcohol can be classified as a food, BUT we need to know that the body does NOT register it as a carbohydrate, protein, or fat. These foods are calorie dense (for the most part) and the calories from alcohol are considered "empty." This is true because alcoholic beverages contain only negligible amounts of vitamins and minerals.

Alcohol is also processed differently than a carbohydrate, protein, or fat. Carbohydrates and protein contain 4 calories per gram, and fat contains 9. Alcohol contains 7 calories per gram. Even though alcohol provides almost twice the calories per gram of either carbohydrates or protein, the good news is it's still less than a gram of fat. So, if you know you're going to be having a glass of wine or two, or a few drinks after work, make sure to factor in those extra calories.

Alcohol can be heart healthy. Having a glass of red wine per day (and no more) can increase the level of high-density lipoproteins (HDL) in the blood. HDL is known as the "good cholesterol" and is responsible for keeping your arteries clear.

I was talking the other day to a friend who enjoys a glass or two of wine a night and considers it an extreme food. Even though a drink is not my choice of extreme food, limits are a hard one.

I realize we all have our vices, whether it's enjoying a fine wine, an after-dinner drink, a delicious dessert, or chips and salsa. It's very possible to fit it into your diet without it affecting your health and wellness. Moderation is key.

Strength Training 101
Day 54

 Diet, cardiovascular training, and strength training are the three components needed to have any success with your health and wellness. All three components must be explored and implemented individually.

Oftentimes the strength training component gets little to no attention compared to cardiovascular training and diet. Today we will squash the BIG LIE that says, "strength training is not essential enough to regularly incorporate into my exercise routine."

Strength training, by definition, is a concerted effort to use resistance or weights to work a muscle group. Being active IS beneficial to the body, BUT it takes a focused effort to work muscles by either using weights or your own body weight to get the benefits of strength training.

A well-designed strength-training program can provide the following benefits:

- Helps to slow down or halt muscle loss that accompanies aging. A typical adult loses about one-half pound of muscle per year after the age of 20, which means you feel less energetic and generally weaker.
- Slows bone loss that accompanies aging, and increases bone density
- Maintains or increases joint flexibility
- Helps to manage or reduce pain from ailments such as arthritis
- Improves fitness variables such as glucose metabolism, blood pressure, muscle strength, endurance, body composition, and even insulin sensitivity
- Improves balance and decreases your risk for injury

Strength training can come in many forms. The most obvious is going to the gym and hitting the weight stack. If you're not a gym person, there are many classes available that are designed for strength training, such as my workouts, Cross Fit, yoga, or others that incorporate weights or body weight.

As you continue to walk out your fitness journey, make sure you have strength training as part of your health and wellness puzzle. You deserve all the benefits health has to offer.

Supply and Demand of Food for Fuel
Day 55

rest day The food we eat is used as energy, but today I'd like to share that even the food we eat has its seasons of supply and demand. Let me explain. The definition of supply and demand is "a theory that explains the interaction between the sellers of a resource and the buyers for that resource."

The theory defines the relationship between the price of a given good or product and the willingness of people to either buy or sell it. The same supply and demand applies to the interaction between us and food. Our "body" is the buyer and "food" is the seller. The relationship between the "Body" and "Food" is determined by what type/amount/quality of food the body is in demand of and the willingness of the mind to choose the right supply.

An example of this supply and demand was my sister's walk through her pregnancies. During pregnancy, she learned the way her body best processed food. Due to her body becoming crowded with a baby, she began to feel uncomfortable when she ate too much. She discovered her body did better eating small amounts. This new way of eating carried over after her deliveries. She is extremely thin due to keeping this habit.

It's been almost 13 years since her last delivery and she still looks the same. A few years ago, she learned she had Hashimoto's Disease (an auto immune disease of the thyroid), so the time came again when her body "demanded" a new supply due to her health. She listened and made those changes, and it's solving problems.

What's the supply and demand your body needs for fuel? How much are you moving? How sedentary are you during the day? How old are you? Constant evaluation is necessary.

Who Told You?
Day 56

rest day These three words are powerful. In order to break free from the voices in our head that hold us back from being our physical best, they must first be mentally identified. Have you ever watched a disturbing movie about child abuse? And in that movie, one day they overcome the odds they were destined for?

On a lighter note, when you were young, did an adult, classmate, teacher, or coach ever say something devastating about you and it stuck with you? And you still think about it today? Well, I'm here to tell you, if it's bad, it's a LIE.

In order to break free from negative self-talk, we must go back and ask ourselves, "Who told me that?" This question isn't to get you to harbor unforgiveness toward a particular person but to instead correct those wrong thoughts about yourself.

Personally, three words have taunted me since a very young age. Fat. White. Ugly. No joke. It seems so silly to even write these words out, but they have led me down a path of eating disorders, baking myself in the sun (to where I'd moan in my sleep), to looking for love in all the wrong places.

Still today, I have to combat those three words and say, "NO! NOT TODAY!"

I'd like to encourage you that it's possible to overcome the LIES of the past. Exercise and eating healthy bring up a lot of inner dialogue about how we feel about ourselves. We must be determined to go way back and ask ourselves the question, "Who told me that?" Correct your negative thinking into a positive way of thinking about yourself.

Walking in freedom is possible; loving ourselves is possible, too.

How to Look Your Best
Day 57

If you're looking for a secret to look your best, there is no secret.

Exercise and good nutrition are very key in helping you look your best. Interestingly, most people focus on nutrition and exercise for better health or for weight loss, but they don't typically think of the positive affects it has on your skin.

Your skincare largely affects the way you look. When you exercise, it positively affects the skin's complexion, glow, and youthful appearance. Exercise gets the blood pumping, helping it to flow more efficiently throughout the body and deliver oxygen and nutrients to the skin, nourishing its cells and keeping it vital. Increased blood flow means flushing wastes and toxins out of the skin.

Have you ever noticed your skin looks clearer and more vibrant after a workout? This is largely due to increasing oxygen and nutrients while flushing out waste via sweat.

Good nutrition positively affects your skin. It's no secret that what you put inside your body is reflected on the outside by how you look. Make sure you're doing everything you can, like drinking your water, because this is a big way to get better skin. Without adequate water, your skin looks dry and weathered. Water plumps up the cells and fills the spaces under your skin, nourishing it and making it look fresh and youthful.

Avoid greasy and deep fried foods. They will clog pores, especially if you don't wash your hands after eating them and then touch your skin. Think about it, your skin is the first thing people see. You can either look refreshed or really bogged down. Every single choice we make toward better health matters.

Your skin tells the truth. I encourage you to look your best. You can constantly better yourself and GLOW, because it surely shows.

Bye Bye Stinking Thinking ... Hello Winner
Day 58

Have you ever had a negative thought about exercising or eating right? Of course you have. A health and wellness journey is HARD. The journey requires constant attention and is high maintenance. You might as well be determined to win in this journey.

You're going to take a lot of falls, so the matter needs to be resolved now. You will win. You'll get back up every single time you fall. Do you know what a winner does? They wipe off their knees after every fall then wash away every single negative thought. Winners get back in the race, ONE MORE TIME. Here are some mental notes for winning.

Strive for a better diet no matter how many times you fail. Continually look at your diet and what you're eating. Make changes where you see fit. If you are susceptible to snacking, keep a piece of fruit or some nuts on hand. Constantly check portion sizes, and make sure each meal contains at least one portion of protein, fruit, and/or vegetables.

Pay close attention to your bad habits. This could be anything from eating too much junk food or drinking too much caffeine to smoking or drinking. Make adjustments to these habits one by one. Some will be easy, while others may take months or maybe years to completely achieve victory, but the sooner you start fighting, the better.

Constantly look for ways to maintain your good qualities. Constantly look for ways to improve your health, too. You don't have time for stinking thinking because you've got a lot of positive work to do. No matter where you are in your journey, you can win. If you've fallen, I encourage you! WE ALL FALL. Simply GET BACK UP ONE MORE TIME. It's always worth it, because you're worth it.

Look Around ... Your Small Army is There
Day 59

If you're a parent, you've experienced the undying love for a child. You can understand wanting your children to be surrounded by friends that are a good influence. If you're not a parent, you can still relate to the power of influential people, but more importantly the support system they can provide.

Have you ever surrounded yourself with the wrong kind of people? If we want the best for our children or loved ones, why would we ever want anything different for ourselves? We need to hang around with people that support and inspire us, people that bring out the best in us. Life is too short to subject ourselves to the Debbie Downers of the world that keep us negative and hopeless.

Most people achieve better results when they're kept accountable. Accountability to others can often provide the motivation needed to ensure we overcome our natural resistance. We know we must exercise if we are to stay in shape, but we often allow other things to crowd it out of our daily lives.

When we find people that support us, we can be more honest with ourselves about our choices. Whereas when we just meander along with no one to keep us in check, we can easily veer off track, justifying all the extras which can result in not making any progress.

We need a healthy environment to run to. As you surround yourself with people who are making a difference by watching and listening, it's guaranteed you'll walk away encouraged every time. I encourage you to look around, my fitness friends. Seek out a small army of people to be your support system.

Whether you have something to give your small army or not, surround yourself with them. Get in their midst. The influence of others is powerful.

Persistence Prevails Perfectly
Day 60

Did you know your individual body has a "perfect place" to be when it comes to your health and wellness? If you're wondering what I mean, let me explain. If you eat too much or too little, your body strives to adapt. If you exercise too much or too little, your body strives to adapt. If you strength train, do anything around your yard, house, or do a recreational activity that requires muscle strength, your body strives to adapt.

Your individual body has a "perfect place" where it's meant to thrive at it's best. If you're in constant pursuit of proper eating and exercising your heart and muscles, your body will bring you to that perfect place of function.

There are two keys to finding your "perfect place."

Persistence is key. In order to learn where your perfect place is, you must begin your quest knowing it will take a continued effort, despite all opposition and difficulty life throws at you. Another truth is no one's exempt from the changes a body goes through as the years go by. These facts must be dealt with by making up your mind now to be persistent and push through to eliminate any questions of quitting.

Prevailing is another key. It's crucial to encourage yourself along the way. You must celebrate the small CURRENT victories. They add up to big victories if you don't lose heart. You must recognize your good choices. Be determined to think good thoughts of yourself and PREVAIL.

Your body is constantly striving for that "perfect place" of function. I encourage you to become a lifetime student of the best foods and exercise that make you feel good. Your body will thank you by constantly looking and feeling its best. I challenge you to remember: persistence prevails perfectly.

Chronic Pain
Day 61

Have you ever heard of the saying, "No pain, no gain?" When the pain of movement produces pain far beyond muscle fatigue or onset soreness, it should grab your attention.

Although it's okay to push yourself until you feel the burn of exercise, it's just as important to know when to stop. Pain is the body's way of telling you that something is wrong. It's important to develop a personal understanding of a healthy pain that could possibly become a chronic pain.

I'd like to touch base on some things that may need your extra attention.

Weather can cause pain: Weather change is a biggie for people over the age of 40, but not so big of a deal for people under 40. When the weather changes it also produces a change in barometric pressure. This barometric pressure change can create joint pain. Joint stiffness decreases when you work out with an extended warmup and proper winter fitness wear.

Rest: It's essential. I've had clients who are getting amazing results but get to a point of exhaustion. Getting the adequate amount of sleep can revive them and actually prepare their body to lose more weight. If you're injured, your doctor will likely prescribe rest for your particular pain. Healing also occurs with rest.

Losing weight can help relieve chronic pain. I've had a lot of new clients begin an exercise regimen with bad knees, back issues, and much more. Months later they discover that their pain has diminished. The actual act of exercise helps chronic pain.

Pain is real. I encourage you to listen to your pain. Many people believe that pain is just something you have to live with. Pain should never be ignored. Let's stay wise and listen to what our bodies are trying to say and obey.

Got Hope?
Day 62

rest day Got hope? I hope so! Hope is needed for all arenas of life. Hope must be the foundation for any attempt to succeed. When the storms of life come, you have to dig deep within. Set your sights forward toward your future with steely eyes, staring into the face of adversity, and keep going.

Despite what your health adversity looks like (maybe an injury, a muscle strain or sprain, an accident, or a distraction), you must have unshakable hope. You can't avoid life's circumstances, but with sure hope, you can meet those circumstances head on.

We must be on guard to counteract elements of health that create hopelessness. Physical pain is a big one. When physical pain attacks your body, the first reaction is to quit exercising. Usually when you put down your exercise shoes, good eating habits walk right out the door, too. Pain is NOT a license to lose hope that you're ever going to reach your goal.

Dealing with human nature can be a hopeless one. It's impatient, selfish, and wants things quickly. A lifestyle of health and wellness success is opposite of what you feel. Make a decision now to be everything you can be, despite your feelings.

Distractions will come. To prevent these distractions it's imperative to have an expectant attitude. Things will work out. It's a must to keep exercise a part of life. I like the phrase "prisoners of hope." Think about it. If you're a prisoner, you have no choice about it; you can't be negative. The other alternative is to be a "prisoner of sedentary blah!" So, when times get tough or you're dealing with disappointment, be determined to dig deep and seek out the good.

I challenge you to be a prisoner of hope, and not sedentary blah.

It Takes Calories to Burn Calories
Day 63

I love this fitness truth! When most people decide to lose weight, they think it's time to start moving more and eating less. There is some truth to that, but we can't neglect that it takes calories to burn calories.

You can look at your metabolism like a fire in a fireplace. When you start a fire in a fireplace, you light the match to a small piece of wood, followed by another small piece of wood. Before long, the big logs take in the heat, then catch fire. The result? You have yourself a nice roaring fire! Well, it's the same for our bodies. If you've made up your mind to lose weight, you must use your calories to your advantage to get your fire roaring (metabolism burning).

It's extremely important to eat to keep your metabolism burning. For your body to simply exist, it takes calories. Basal metabolic rate (BMR) is the baseline calorie amount you need to support body functions like breathing and heart rate. In other words, it describes the number of calories you need to survive at rest.

Your BMR is determined by factors such as your gender, age, height, and weight. Everyone has a different BMR. You may have a BMR of 1200 calories per day just to simply exist. A big muscle dude may need 2500 calories per day to exist. I think it's a good reminder that we are burning calories constantly all day long, just from simple body functions.

The human body is much more complex than we realize. Our common goal should be to eat and train most efficiently for our individual bodies. Remember, it takes calories to burn calories. We only have one body; we can't go buy a new one. We might as well treat it well!! :)

Now Why Do I Have to Drink Water?
Day 64

Drinking water is one of the healthiest things you can do for better wellness. I talk a lot about water, because it's very important. Drinking eight cups a day is beneficial. Drinking this daily quota increases fat reduction, enhances healthier skin, gives you more energy, and can even help with better digestion.

Here are some tips in meeting your daily quota:

Invest in a water bottle. Splurge on the perfect reusable water bottle. Whether it's your favorite color or a unique design, the more you bond with your bottle, the more likely you'll want to use it. You could even decorate your bottle.

Sip it. Gulping it only shoots the water straight through your digestive tract with little to no absorption. Sipping your water will allow your body the time it needs to absorb it into your bloodstream.

Become a connoisseur. Think of water drinking like wine tasting. Taste the various brands and types of bottled waters available (sparkling, spring, mineral, vitamin-enhanced, filtered, fruit-flavored, etc.). Be sure to read the labels, as some "waters" have significantly added calories.

Drink and drive. Keep your water bottle next to you every time you hop into the car, or buy a package of bottled water to keep in the car. Whenever you're driving about, your water will be within easy reach from your car's cup holder.

Drink your vitamins. Create your own vitamin drink. Consider combining your water with your vitamin supplements (if you take them). There are several powdered vitamin supplements that are designed to be mixed with water.

Drinking water can be made fun and simple. Cultivating a water habit will only make you healthier. Our bodies are mostly made up of water. Water is a vital component for body function. I challenge you to drink up.

How Much Do You Weigh?
Day 65

How much do you weigh? What a question. No one likes to talk about how much they weigh, especially ladies. Both my young adolescent girls came to me and asked the question, "How much SHOULD I weigh?" Another time, I was eavesdropping on a conversation (of a group of kids) asking each other how much they weighed. It grieved me to think how much you weigh is such a big deal to the youth.

I've always wondered who came up with the so called "perfect weight" and how it's associated with being pretty or looking good. It's important to know body weight and composition are two different things. Weight is a unit of mass (as in a pound or kilogram). Body composition means the fat-to-muscle ratio of your body.

People get hung up on a scale number and ignore body composition. Weight loss is somewhat meaningless unless you talk about body composition. For instance, you could have a 250-pound male body builder that has 5 percent body fat and is one solid muscle. Or you could have a 250-pound male with a 50% overall fat percentage that would obviously need to make some changes toward weight loss. Therefore, the scale number "250" does NOT need to be the focus; body composition does.

Everyone fluctuates. I have a doctor friend who told me once the weight charts in a doctor's office aren't even medically backed. Doctor's office weight charts are actually designed by an insurance company. My fit doctor friend does NOT refer to those charts, but encourages his clients to eat healthy and exercise regularly if they exceed the recommended weight according to his charts.

It's no one's business how much you weigh. Set your focus on the things that produce true health and wellness.

You've Got This
Day 66

Not long ago, you were energetic and determined to begin a healthy lifestyle. Starting with enthusiasm and hope, you watched your food intake diligently and exercised faithfully. You were confident to reach your goals once and for all! Then the mundaneness of it all set in. You ate an extra piece of cake. You missed a workout, which turned into a whole week away from exercising. Your momentum to start over again is gone. Does this sound familiar?

What do you do? I'll tell you what to do. GET UP. It's never too late. I like to look at fitness like mountains and valleys. Mountain experiences are awesome, but unfortunately no one can stay there. There are valleys in everyone's journey.

If you find your momentum slipping, you're probably experiencing a valley. When you're in a valley there are two choices. Stay where you are, and find yourself even further away from your goals; or accept your lack of perfection, forgive yourself, and do the next right thing.

You've never messed up beyond the point of no return. Start TODAY.

Here are some suggestions to help you when the "healthy stuff" seems overwhelming.

- Try a short workout. Five minutes is better than nothing. Take a walk.
- Try a new recipe. Healthy foods can taste delicious; have fun trying some.
- Eat a healthy breakfast. Begin your day with a good food choice.
- Observe and listen to how others overcome their struggles and obstacles; it's motivating.
- Share your goals. Accountability is powerful. Get support from friends.
- Create a motivational collage. Include pictures of your goals and reasons why you want to get there.

If you expect perfection, you're setting yourself up for disappointment. Health and wellness journeys are messy. There is no better day than today. You've got this.

Do You Have Proper Underwear?
Day 67

When you were leaving home as a teenager, did your momma ever tell you to not forget your underwear since you never know when you might get in a wreck? Well, as we have aged, we have all learned that underwear is extremely important. This fact is especially true when exercising.

A sports bra is essential. Sports bras give support to reduce bounce and uncomfortable motion. They are designed to move well as you twist and bend. When choosing a good sports bra, make sure it's breathable (made with sweat-wicking fabric rather than cotton). The sweat-wicking fabric will help prevent chafing. As for the men, a sweat-wicking fitted undershirt will prevent the common nipple chafing that occurs with avid runners and such.

Underwear for both men and women need to be moisture-wicking with breathable fabrics. In deciding on the shape and style, be experimental. Exercise can increase irritation from underwear; pick a smooth fabric rather than lace, designs, or trims. Many exercise shorts have there own built-in liner that doesn't require underwear, always a comfortable choice. Again, these are recommendations, but you'll be the deciding factor through experimentation.

The ultimate goal here is to prevent skin irritation and risk of infection. If you experience any discomfort with your undergarments, it probably won't get any better. You can chalk that discomfort up as experimental and try another undergarment. If you have a friend that has a similar body type, ask for their suggestions. I've found the greatest success in asking advice about clothes from my fitness family.

It's a good reminder to remember your underwear is just as important or maybe even more important than what you wear to exercise in!

I Don't Want to Get Bulky
Day 68

We all have an idea in our head when it comes to looking our fittest and healthiest. For some of us, it's fitting perfectly into a certain outfit, or walking on the beach in a bikini with total confidence. For others, it's striving for a defined midsection, or having strong, toned shoulders or legs.

Our specific goals differ in how we want to look and feel. In helping people reach their goals, I hear statements like, "I want to be toned, not bulky," or "every time I lift weights I feel so bulky." Let's clarify the difference between toned and bulky.

What does toned mean? Toning is a term used to describe the end goal, which usually results from a combination of basic weightlifting and fat burning. When most people say that they want to "tone up," what they usually mean is that they want to become leaner. They want to lose fat and add a little muscle definition.

What does bulking up mean? "Bulking up" means adding a lot of muscle mass to the body and possibly (although not always) reducing one's body fat, too. Bulking up usually brings the images of bodybuilders or big football players. We usually think of a male that has big, bulging muscles! Typically, men want to "bulk up" and women usually want to avoid building big, bulky muscles.

Don't be afraid to lift weights. When you do, make sure you are using a weight that is heavy enough that the last two repetitions are challenging to lift. Only then is the body challenged enough to change, grow, and adapt. The beauty of weightlifting is it's making you stronger and leaner no matter if you're male or female, old or young. Lifting weights tones ALL bodies well.

Constructive Conflict
Day 69

rest day

When the word "conflict" is spoken, usually it's not used in a positive light. The definition of conflict is "to come into collision or disagreement; be contradictory, at variance, or in opposition; clash; a fight, battle, or struggle, especially a prolonged struggle; strife." Most of us avoid any sense of the word, but when it pertains to exercise and growth, or reaching the next level, conflict is a good thing.

As you want to grow or begin exercising regularly, you must know from the start you'll face physical conflict. The two words in the definition above that apply to fitness are battle and struggle.

Let's discuss these two words to have a better understanding.

Exercise is a battle. It's a battle physically and mentally. There's a battle during each workout. It begins with showing up, then comes the training, the knowing that you're going to sweat, experiencing labored breathing, and impatiently wanting class over.

Exercise is a struggle by not knowing what to expect. The very act of getting to the gym is "a struggle;" knowing you're going to struggle doing what your workout requires; knowing that the struggle will be worth it because no one ever regrets completing a workout.

I have a precious client that comes to class every time saying, "I'm on the struggle bus."

She shows up faithfully and accepts the battle and struggle of exercise. The constructive conflict fitness brings will produce results. My client produces results.

Have you ever heard of the saying, "The very thing that elms you, is the very thing you need?" Let's all be those people that go after whatever it takes. A lover of fitness craves each workout and has their own personal, constructive way of creating conflict. I challenge you to seek your very own constructive conflict.

Being Active Pyramid Style
Day 70

I'd like to share a written visual of what an active lifestyle looks like in a pyramid form, broken into four sections. Visualize a pyramid divided horizontally in four rows. I'm here to show you that a little exercise in all four categories goes a long way. Let's work from the top down.

The top section represents activities that burn the least amount of calories. You should be spending the least time watching T.V., playing video games, etc. (sitting no more than 30 minutes at a time).

The next section from the top of the pyramid: Recreational activities like golf, bowling, and archery, or muscle exercises like stretching or weightlifting (2-3 times per week).

The third section from top of the pyramid: Recreational activities like football, tennis, basketball, or dancing (for at least 30 minutes duration) or aerobic activity (swimming, running, biking, or skiing for at least 20 minutes duration 3-5 times a week).

The bottom section of the pyramid: Walking the dog or walking with a friend, taking the stairs, gardening, or parking the farthest from the supermarket (daily, done leisurely).

Chose one activity from each pyramid section to create an active lifestyle.

Here's my sample active lifestyle:

- Top section of the pyramid: I love my Netflix.
- Next section of the pyramid from the top: I lift weights five days a week.
- The third section from the top: I bike 5 times a week for 50-60 minutes.
- Bottom section of the pyramid: I either walk my dog or walk with a friend.

I hope this visual helps bring understanding to a healthy lifestyle. If you're not even close to any of these activities, receive this as encouragement. This is a great model on how to get started by offering different things that you can do.

Sedentary -
Watching TV, Sitting
Less than 30 minutes at a time

Recreational Activities: Golf, Bowling, Archery
Muscle Exercises: Stretching or Weightlifting
2-3 times per week

Recreational Activities: Football, Tennis, Basketball, Dancing
Aerobic Activities: Swimming, Running, Biking, Skiing
3-5 times per week for at least 20 minutes

Leisure Activities: Walking the dog, Walking with a friend, Taking the
Stairs, Gardening, Parking farthest from buildings
Daily at your Leisure

Enjoying the Journey is a ... MUST
Day 71

Stepping on the elliptical machine the other morning, I dug down deep for some motivation. It seemed harder for some reason. Frustrating, disappointing, hopeless, and skeptical thoughts filled my mind as I had an hour and a half workout ahead. When my workout came to an end, I felt great, but I quickly thought back to how I felt beforehand. I realized those emotions are common enemies of people trying to lose weight or improve themselves. You must seek enjoyment in the journey.

You've got to keep in mind that exercise always boosts your self-esteem, confidence, and happiness. When you're committed to a weekly exercise routine, you feel more comfortable in your own body. Be determined to build a positive vocabulary to stay motivated and cast down any emotion that tries to keep you from exercising regularly.

Expect to find unexpected joy. Allow yourself to expect to be happier and to experience more vibrancy, excitement, and enjoyment. All healthy emotions are well worth the workout. The unexpected joy could even be a better night's sleep or to be more focused. Start listening to the signs your body gives you that all your hard work is paying off. Tap into the unexpected joys.

Exercise is so personal; we all have very different dreams and aspirations. Personal disappointments vary vastly. You can find understanding in a fitness family. They can help you overcome disappointing hurtles. Enjoy your fitness family; you may even laugh in the process.

I encourage you to enjoy the good things that are going on inside and outside your body. Enjoy your mobility and independence. It's never a wrong choice to exercise. Remember exercise is your antidote. ENJOY YOURSELF.

Endurance through Perseverance
Day 72

There are two words that need to be a BIG part of your health and wellness: endurance and perseverance. The definition of endurance is the ability or strength to continue or last especially despite fatigue, stress, or other adverse conditions. Perseverance is defined as persistence in the course of action even in the face of difficulty or with little or no prospect of success.

When you initially get started toward better health, you feel motivated and encouraged. Usually friends and family get on board to cheer you on because they're happy for you. Then comes those ordinary days, and it's just you with no one around to cheer you on. Then it becomes easier to skip those days and just go home.

That is easy to do when no one is around. Your new fitness success is now old news, and you're tired and bored with it, and simply want to call it a day. Right there…right at that particular moment … is when you must pull up that word "endurance" from the back of your brain and let the positive self-talk begin.

Self-talk goes something like this, "Yes, I'm tired and bored, and no one really cares if I'm ten pounds lighter, BUT, I WILL drum up the strength. I'll go work out despite how I'm feeling. I know it will help my fatigue, stress, and mood, and then I can go home and lay on the couch and actually enjoy it guilt-free."

You must remember wherever your mind goes your body will surely follow. So, you must persevere when adverse conditions arise. Don't be tempted to give up. Endure and persevere and you'll find the encouragement and motivation you need to keep going.

Money-Back Guarantee
Day 73

Have you ever bought fitness equipment or anything that comes with a money-back guarantee? The manufacturer is confident you WILL achieve results if you do as instructed. To be the best you can be physically, however, you must work in three different categories. These are resistance training which is weight lifting or weight bearing exercises, cardiovascular training which is continued movement of any sort that keeps your heart rate elevated over any extended period of time, and diet which is the biggest one to conquer. Below are some ways to get maximum results in each area.

To get maximum results in strength training, your goal is to get a well-rounded, balanced workout. You can achieve this by hiring a personal trainer or training with me. My videos, posted Monday through Friday, are designed to train all muscle groups weekly which meets that goal.

To get maximum results in cardiovascular training, you should exercise four to six days each week. These days should be spread throughout the week and not done all at once. We call people who exercise all at once "weekend warriors" because they take it easy during the week and train hard on the weekends. This is a dangerous way of exercising because it adds extra stress to your heart. Instead of doing two hard workout days and five rest days, the weekend warrior would benefit from exercising each of the five weekdays and resting on the weekends.

To get maximum results in your diet, you can hire a registered dietitian. You can also educate yourself and learn all you can about your body and how it responds to the particular foods you eat.

I challenge you to implement all three categories in your journey. It works, and that I can guarantee.

Three-Stage Cycle of Fitness
Day 74

I was in Atlanta the other day and needed to set the GPS in intimidating traffic, knowing I had to get the address right or I would be really lost. As I began my route, I thought of exercise. There comes a time in all our fitness pursuits when we must be precise about where we're going or we'll get lost.

There's a three-stage cycle of fitness that must be completed before adopting exercise as a lifestyle.

The first stage: Getting started. This is the hardest stage because it's so emotional. We have such high hopes in what we want out of exercise. When we don't get exactly what we want when we want it, we get downright angry, frustrated, sad, and close to giving up. In order to get started, there needs to be a learning curve in discovering what works for you.

The second stage: Setting your GPS. Let's say you found my YouTube videos or CrossFit as your new passion for fitness. Take time to figure out your precise schedule for the week and don't vary.

The third stage: Doing your routine until it's time to revisit. Imagine years have gone by. You're as fit as a fiddle from following your regimen. There isn't anything that is going to get in your way of a workout at this point … then … BOOM. Some kind of body pain arises or an injury occurs that places you in physical therapy. Now you have to revisit your fitness routines. Here's where the going gets tough. Something you've done for years without even thinking about is now in desperate need of change. This is the time to use the three-stage cycle to get you going in a new direction.

I challenge you to think about what stage you're in.

How Can I Improve My Core Strength?
Day 75

Today I'd like to share three progressive moves that can easily be done to improve your core strength. These specific exercises are designed to progress safely while at the same time sculpt a flat, strong midsection.

Here are the three core moves.

Progression 1: Lie on your back. Knees are bent and feet are flat on the floor. Hips are level and the spine is sinking into the floor as if it's a sandbox. Shoulders are pressed back and down toward your buttocks. Now, lift legs, feet toward the ceiling, arms extended out to the side creating the letter T. Inhale. Then as you exhale, press your arms toward the ground for support as you lift your bottom off the ground. Now for a count of six, bring your legs toward the floor. Reverse the motion for a count of six, back to the starting position. Repeat 20 reps (3 sets).

Progression 2: Use the same starting position as Progression 1. This time your feet face the wall, legs creating a 90-degree angle at your knees and hips. Keep the shoulder blades down, using the same resistance as before. Inhale. Then, as you exhale, bring your bent legs to the right side (hold for six counts), back to the center, then bring your bent legs to the left side (hold for six counts). Repeat 20 reps (3 sets).

Progression 3: Combine both exercises above for 20 reps (3 sets).

Your mid-section is a combination of small, stabilizer muscles, not large muscles. To experience the best results, I challenge you to eat a healthy diet alongside your core work. Don't be fooled by the simplicity! Adding these three progression core exercises can do great things. Be encouraged.

No Formula for Fitness
Day 76

rest day We're never supposed to assume, but in this case, I'm pretty sure it's okay to assume that we all like formulas that will bring answers. Over the years of helping people attain their fitness goals, one common theme is they all want "the" diet and "the" fitness plan to get them where they desire to go. I truly wish I had that magic formula to give all my clients that are seeking better health.

The hard truth is, there is no formula for fitness. We all desire optimal health in this world that tells us there is some magic pill or diet or fitness routine formula. No amount of money can buy that perfect formula, because it doesn't exist.

The human body is wonderfully multifaceted. We all are very different. We all have specific needs, restrictions, and desires. In these differences, there is great beauty. Our goals are different. Each vision is different. Even each day is different. Going into our own individual fitness journey, we must not confuse formulas with plans.

Formulas are fiction but plans are reality. You plan by setting small goals and crossing them off as you go. This is guaranteed success. Your fitness dreams can come true by setting those goals. Dreaming of better fitness without any goals only leads to frustration. My clients that are goal-oriented reap rewards.

I encourage you as you exercise today to stay consistent with your plan. By golly, take your commitment to exercise in one hand and your plan to get there in the other, and nothing will stop your success. Be determined to bulldoze forward and watch the sparks fly. Squash the lie of that magic formula. It doesn't exist. You will enjoy your life of planning for success!

Protein Powders
Day 77

rest day

Have you ever wondered what all the hype is about protein powders? Why is almost everyone in the gym carrying around these funny looking bottles with this powder substance in them?

What exactly is protein powder? It's a substance that is made up of nine amino acids that equals a complete protein necessary for human dietary needs. You can have a protein drink and get the complete protein that your body needs for proper recovery and growth.

Do you need to implement protein powder in your diet? Maybe.

Here are a few reasons why the ordinary athlete might want more protein in his or her diet:

When you are growing. A teenager needs more protein to fuel his workouts because his body is still growing and uses more protein.

When you are starting a workout program. If working out is new to you and you're trying to build muscle, you'll require more protein than normal.

When you're adding more intensity to your workouts. If you work out for thirty minutes a few times a week, but now you've decide to train for a half-marathon, your body will need more protein.

When you're recovering from an injury. Athletes with sports injuries frequently need more protein to help them heal.

When to supplement protein powders? If you calculate your protein intake and determine you're not getting enough for your athletic needs, adding a protein powder is good.

How can you best use protein powders to help you improve your performance? Experiment before, during, or after your workouts and determine your peak performance.

Adding protein powders could be just what you need in catapulting you to a new fitness level. It could be what your body needs to strengthen your immune system. I encourage you to try protein today.

Doing Something New Produces ... Results
Day 78

Yes - Results. I bet I have your attention. We all want them and want them now. An individual's health is a very personal thing. I respect the many different ways to attain fitness success. But today let's talk about the similarities in getting results from our journeys. There are three similarities that need attention.

Underestimating your eating. Many people are in denial about the foods they eat, particularly about the quantities consumed. If you really want to lose weight, you need to be honest with yourself about what you put into your mouth and how that helps or hinders your weight-loss goals.

Overestimating your exercise. Most exercisers are far too generous with estimates of exercise intensity and time, the amount of weight lifted, and the frequency of their workouts. To avoid overestimation, it's helpful to keep an exercise log and track these items initially. I'm not a big chart person, but writing things down in the beginning will help show you exactly where you stand and how to make changes more easily.

Never changing your workout. A plateau is just around the corner. Change is hard but it's a must for results. When you do the same thing day after day, you get very good at it. In exercise, this is called the principle of adaptation. It basically means that you become very efficient by doing the same exercise over and over. This is great for sports performance, but not that great for weight loss, increasing strength, or physical fitness progression. One way of overcoming this plateau is to modify your workouts every few weeks or months.

Results are attainable. Why do they seem so hard to achieve? It's because they're not for the weak at heart. Don't let go until you see the results.

Almond Butter -vs- Peanut Butter
Day 79

A client once asked me, "Why is almond butter better for you than peanut butter?" After comparing the two in response to her question, I thought it worth the time to share my reasoning with you as to why I think almond butter should be a staple in your pantry.

When it comes to nut butters, it's hard to beat peanut butter in popularity. I learned 90% of the kitchen cabinets in the United States stock peanut butter on their shelves. While peanut butter is a healthy choice as far as nut butters go, there are good reasons to consider buying almond butter, too.

One, almond butter is richer in heart-healthy fats. Almond butter is a slightly better source, with 5 grams per tablespoon versus 3.3 grams per tablespoon in peanut butter.

Two, it is also a slightly better source of fiber. One tablespoon of almond butter contains 1.6 grams of fiber while peanut butter has 0.9 grams. Most Americans don't get enough fiber in their diet and do not meet their daily fiber needs.

Three, it is a significant source of vitamin E. As a matter of fact, it has four times more vitamin E than peanut butter. Vitamin E is a fat-soluble vitamin known for its antioxidant properties.

Four, almond butter has more minerals. Minerals such as calcium, iron, potassium, and zinc are essential nutrients your body needs to function properly. When comparing the two nut butters, almond butter is a better source of these minerals.

All in all, almond butter is more nutritious than peanut butter. It may be more expensive, but nowadays, peanut butter is getting more expensive, too. I encourage you to vary your diet and consider making almond butter a part of your weekly eating plan.

Just Don't Do It
Day 80

Just don't do it. It sounds so simple, but when it comes to over-eating, it's not that simple. I've talked about binge eating before, but I believe it's a topic worth revisiting. Binge eating is a disorder, which requires treatment - not the words "Just don't do it."

Two-thirds struggling with a binge-eating disorder are overweight. People who binge feel bad about their weight. This leads to low self-esteem, which usually causes more overeating. The good news is there are solutions. One solution is to figure out why you're overeating. Your doctor or a therapist can help you get started. Another solution is talk to a dietitian and come up with a diet and exercise program you can stick with.

Binge eating makes your heart work a lot harder and makes it more difficult for your heart to pump blood to the lungs and body. Eating excessive amounts of food all at once raises your risk of high blood pressure, high cholesterol, and high blood sugar. All of these things boost your risk for heart attack and stroke. You might also need medicine to lower your blood pressure, cholesterol, and blood sugar to regulate you while you're working on eating properly.

Depression and anxiety are more common in people with binge eating disorder. A lot of people who binge eat do so to boost their mood. This can lead to guilty feelings that just make you binge more. One solution I've found is exercise. Exercising releases a 'feel good' chemical, serotonin, which is a mood-altering chemical.

Food should give us energy and enhance our daily lives. Food should NOT give you bad digestion problems or make you feel like you have to take a nap or unbutton your pants. You're better than binge eating. There's hope.

Opportunity for Gain, Not Loss
Day 81

Have you ever reflected on your past? No one is exempt from struggles. I'm sure you've had struggles. Most of the time you can get stuck looking in the past of loss and forget there are a lot of good things to gain. I'd like to focus on what you can do for GAIN during the present day and not LOSS of the past.

Have you ever heard a person's perception is their current reality? What's been your daily FOCUS? If your focus is gloom and doom, let's begin by focusing on taking care of yourself and your loved ones. Let's begin with basic fitness and nutrition. The outdoors bring healing. A simple short walk will enlighten you in ways you didn't think possible. If your struggle is overeating, pray about it. Pray for a new perspective and a new reality, and use it for gain. I pray daily about my struggle with food. One morning, I thought to myself, boy I'm getting sick and tired of praying about this. Then suddenly, my thoughts switched over to choosing to change my perception and creating a new reality.

You have a choice. It's true. We all have choices. You can use your current situation as an opportunity. Exercise the action to love, be joyful, and seek peace in all your new situations to be patient with yourself and others. Your loved ones need you healthy with a perception of good gain for a bright future.

Respond to stressful things with kindness. Find an opportunity to be good to yourself and others. Continue to be faithful and diligent in doing what needs to be done. I challenge you to go forward into this new season and perceive new realities for opportunities to gain in life and not look back at loss.

In It To Win It
Day 82

There are a million and one ways to keep your weight under control. I had a client just the other day (who has lost 19 pounds and is still going strong) share her story. I wish I could say it was profound advice, but it wasn't. She discovered some small ways to win. Her simple words of success were, "It all boils down to portion control and exercise."

I'd like to share some minor nutritional adjustments she used to help with portion control.

She served her dinner on individual plates. She left the extra food on the stove. It takes about 20 minutes for your mind to get the signal from your belly that you are full. So, bowls of food on the table beg to be eaten, and it takes incredible willpower to not dig in for seconds.

She started eating slowly. She made it a goal to chew every bite and savored the taste of her meal. She also put down her fork between bites and drank plenty of water with her meals.

She stopped eating a snack after dinner and brushed her teeth afterwards to help fight the temptation of eating again.

She started eating breakfast. She found that she wasn't as hungry when lunch rolled around, so she could practice more self-control at lunch. Breakfast is the most important meal of the day. After a long night's rest, your body needs the fuel to get your metabolism going and give you energy for the rest of the day.

We're in our health and wellness to win. Weight control is all about making small changes that you can live with forever. I challenge you to find ways you can make some nutritional adjustments or even to try one my client's practices.

Mental Health
Day 83

rest day

In the beginning, we dive into the fitness arena to improve our exterior appearance, but what we soon learn is our mental health improves, too. Most people who exercise regularly continue to do so because it gives them an enormous sense of well-being. They feel more energetic throughout the day, sleep better at night, have sharper memories, feel more relaxed, and are more positive about themselves.

Exercise is a powerful medicine for many common mental health challenges such as depression, trauma, and post-traumatic stress disorder. It promotes all kinds of changes in the brain, including neural growth, reduced inflammation, and new activity patterns that promote feelings of calmness and well-being. When we focus on how our bodies feel as we exercise, our nervous systems can become unstuck, allowing us to move out of the immobilizing response of trauma.

Exercise also helps manage stress. When under stress, our muscles get tense especially those in our faces, necks, and shoulders, which can cause back and neck pain and painful headaches. We can feel a tightness in our chests, pounding heartbeats, and muscle cramps in our limbs. Other health problems such as insomnia, heartburn, stomachache, diarrhea, and frequent urination may also occur. The worry and discomfort of these physical symptoms can in turn cause even more stress, thus creating a vicious cycle between our minds and bodies.

Exercising is an effective way to break this cycle. Since the body and mind are so closely linked, when our bodies feel better so do our minds. Regular exercising is one of the easiest and most effective ways to reduce stress symptoms and to improve concentration, motivation, memory, and mood. These are wonderful mental health benefits. Quitting exercise prematurely is not an option. Exercise is for a lifetime.

Whey Protein
Day 84

rest day

Now you know that there are two major proteins, casein and whey. Whey protein is the building block that provides protein and amino acids for increased muscle growth. Whey protein is the more common protein that is recommended for consumption after a workout.

Casein protein is a slow-digesting protein, whereas whey is a fast-digesting protein. Fast digesting means the amount of time it takes to be fully metabolized. This is why it's recommended to be taken right after a workout. It is quickly absorbed into the blood, absorbed by bodily tissues, and completes one of many metabolic facets.

Upon ingestion, it takes only 20 minutes before almost all of what you have consumed is coursing through your veins. This is why in the gym you see "big guys" or the "serious fitness competitors" carrying around their bottle shakers and drinking their protein ASAP.

Some benefits of adding whey to your diet:

Muscle growth is dependent on the balance between protein synthesis and breakdown. If the synthesis of new muscle protein (which is your added whey protein powder) is greater than the breakdown of muscle protein (which comes from training), net gains in muscle mass are seen.

Fat loss and preserve muscle. Studies have proven that those consuming whey lost a significantly greater amount of body fat and better preserved their muscles. If you have an urge to snack on something, a great alternative is to try a whey drink or shake.

Increase strength and size. Studies have also proven that those who consumed whey had greater increases in fat-free muscle mass and strength.

In making protein a priority, you will be pleased with the results of how well your muscles respond to your workouts. So, cheers ... drink up ... protein does the body good. :)

Who Are Your Friends?
Day 85

If you're a parent, I'm sure you've been concerned about the friends your children are hanging around. Maybe you're a son or daughter and you've heard your mom or dad say, "I don't like who you're hanging out with; they're not a good influence." Why should it be any different for adults?

We truly do become who we hang out with. Even as adults, we can still be greatly influenced by others' actions. Did you know by observing the five closest people in your life, you'll see the kind of person you are or will become within 5 years? Within those particular people, is at least one of the five someone you can look up to, learn from, and be challenged by?

Does at least one encourage you to be a better parent, worker, or friend? When we're seeking better health and wellness, we must first take a look at the main influences in our lives. Do you have at least one or two within your immediate five closest friends that challenge you to grow in your health and wellness and are willing to hold you accountable for your betterment?

Having the right friends helps to keep you in the right mindset. The way you think drives your actions, so surround yourself with positive friends that keep you encouraged on the days that you'd rather just go home. This also works both ways. You can be their encouragement on the days they want to throw in the towel and go home.

If you find that your closest friends aren't the best influences, try to make new ones by venturing and finding fitness friends to glean from. Possibilities are always endless. I encourage you to get your hopes up and never give up.

Do the Next Right Thing
Day 86

Home quarantine was challenging and got old quick. Growing weary in doing what needed to be done was experienced by most of us. Working from home, homeschooling kids, not being able to do the simple errands for your family, etc. These are some legit things to grow weary from.

I have good news (even post quarantine) on a healthy way to handle this new norm we're facing. I've sat in a counseling chair pretty much most of my life and learned the best way to handle things that are too profound for me is to do the next right thing. We all have our particular environments. Look around you. What is your job? How old are your kids? How old are your parents? Where exactly are you in life?

A healthy outlet for all the answers above is to EXERCISE and DON'T WORRY. Facing the unknown is the new norm now. During this "new norm" we get the opportunity to "do the next right thing" with a positive mindset. One of my favorite scriptures that has helped me handle things that are too profound for me is Philippians 4:8: "Finally, brothers and sisters, whatever is true, whatever is noble, whatever is right, whatever is pure, whatever is lovely, whatever is admirable – if anything is excellent or praiseworthy – think about such things."

Make exercise your next right thing. Exercising is something that's in your control during this time. It's easier to find the bad. Let's be determined to find hidden blessings. We all have blessings in our lives. I challenge you to do your job with outstanding, superior quality. Praise GOD for your job and your health. Let's make the best of this post-quarantine life by not growing weary and doing the next right thing.

Finding Joy in the Journey
Day 87

You've got to make health and wellness a lifestyle for sustaining success. It's true. You must find some kind of continual movement with a healthy way of eating, then apply it to most days of your week to achieve lasting results.

When you think of the word "exercise," what comes to mind? Dread or joy? When I take on a new client, my biggest goal is to help them find JOY. A telltale sign of clients finding that joy (or I call it crossing over to the other side) is when they have to miss a workout in the afternoon but wake up first thing the next morning to make up for what they missed.

Exercise becomes a mission that must be completed. There's no longer dread associated with exercise; it's either something always good or extremely satisfying upon completion.

Joy can look different to each individual. Here are two different categories: good and satisfying.

Good category:
- You find joy in the hard work of exercise.
- You find joy in the sweat.
- You find joy in the burn.
- You find joy in the soreness of a workout brought on from a couple of days earlier.
- You find joy in almost having to throw up but not.

Satisfying category:
- You find joy completing the class or style of fitness you love.
- You find joy in having your friend work out with you.
- You find joy in the extra energy your workout brings.
- You find joy in learning that you're stronger and need heavier weights.
- You find joy in meeting a set goal.

Whatever kind of joy you can find about exercise, cling to it. All of the above are real life testimonies of clients over the years, sharing how they find joy. I encourage you to find enJOYment in your journey.

Discovery, Discovery, and More Discovery
Day 88

Do you want me to let you in on a big truth? Exercise is for YOU.

I didn't say the SAME exercise is for everyone. As individuals, we must go out into this big world of fitness and find what works for us. One big aspect of this truth is discovery. We all must have a body awareness that leads to constant discovery. Then you can adapt accordingly.

Here are some examples of discovery and how to adapt. I'll use personal experiences and other stories that have taught me over the years.

My first discovery was the food amount that I could consume changed as the years went by. I discovered that as I got older, I could no longer consume large amounts of food. I've had to adapt accordingly.

My second discovery was that as we age we lose muscle mass. I've had to adapt by not training with heavy weights as I did in the past. I have a client who loves basketball, but the agility it takes to play was causing him minor injuries. Mind you, he was really good at basketball, but his big discovery was to hang up those basketball shoes before a major injury occurred.

My third discovery was aches and pains that take place as we age. I had a client that ran a 5k with her daughter. She discovered new knee pain. She wasn't sure if it was from weight gain or age. She didn't allow her aches and pains to be a reason for complaining, but instead she discovered to adapt in ways her body needed.

Awareness is wisdom, so listen to your body. You must always be open to discovering new responses of your body and learn how to adapt accordingly.

Goal Setters
Day 89

 It's important to find people in your circle of influence that are goal setters, people who desire and plan to do something significant with their lives, people who are going to help you become all that the good Lord created you to be.

We all have something unique that only we are designed to do. These visions take a healthy body to execute. That is why health and wellness goals are essential. The Bible says, "A man without a vision shall perish. Write the vision and make it plain on tablets, so that the one who reads it may run with it."

This should encourage you to discover your fitness goals, write them down, and GO FOR IT.

You must begin small. I have a precious client that reports to me every month. She writes down her goals, then sends them to me. This is great for two reasons. First, she constantly has a fresh new plan in play, and second, she is accountable to me. She reevaluates her strengths and weaknesses at the beginning of every month then tweaks her existing plan accordingly. The best part of this story is her success has been AMAZING.

You must have long-term goals. You should have those big dreams and goals for yourself, but a plan to get there must be explored. Making a map of short-term goals to achieve our long-term goals is the answer. With your long-term vision before you, walking out these baby steps one foot at a time keeps you motivated to achieve your ultimate dreams.

I realize this information may seem very elementary, but believe it or not, people forget the simplicity of it all. Every dream you have, write it down. Find people with similar goals and dreams. Surround yourself with greatness!!

SECOND QUARTER
Daily Inspirations for Fitness

Moving Right Along
Days 90-180

**Scan the QR Code for each day
to take you to a companion
YouTube Video Workout**

Are You Led by Purpose or Desire?
Day 90

rest day

Desire is wonderful. Desires are aspirations about wishes and wants. Someone once told me if wishes and wants were donuts and money, we'd all be fat and rich!

We've all got desires and dreams. The problem is that desires don't mean anything until we purpose or determine in our heart to make them a reality. To have "purpose" means to have tenacity and drive; to be resolute about a quest; to be so driven that you won't let anything get in your way.

Desires can be used in helping you achieve your fitness, health, and wellness goals. For example, if you desire to run a marathon, then purpose it in your heart to do so. Set a goal, train, and do it.

If you have no specific desire but generally want to get active or remain active, then it's your job to begin each day purposing in your heart to do what is profitable. Set reachable goals and don't be led astray by whimsical desires that may keep you from a life of victory.

I challenge you to purpose daily to:

• Exercise four days out of a seven-day week.

• Eat something good one day a week, then two days a week, then three days a week, etc.

• Don't go solo; find friends that love healthy ways of living.

• Don't let bad news or bad weather stop you. Exercise can be a great, healthy, constructive distraction.

• Don't let the "I just want to go home" syndrome get in your way. Exercising beforehand makes going home that much more pleasurable.

I encourage you to make sure your desires are backed by purpose. To purpose is to have drive. To purpose is to take action. To purpose is to achieve victory!

Time Killer or Time Filler
Day 91

rest day   What do you consider as a good way to spend your time? Have you ever walked away from doing something and said to yourself, "I'm so glad I did that," or "I hate I did that?" Here are a few examples of what I mean.

- Eating with a friend (glad I did that) but I overate (hate I did that).
- Went to happy hour with coworkers for one glass of wine (glad I did that) but stayed and had three more glasses (hate I did that).
- Shopped with family (glad I did that) but spent way over my budget (hate I did that).
- Got invited to walk with friends but chose the buffet instead (hate I did that); a new friend invited me to try a new fitness class, and I joined her (glad I did that).

As you can see from these examples, we often fill our time with "good" time fillers and "not so good" time killers.

It's good to look forward a bit to make a plan for utilizing good time fillers in order to avoid bad time killers. By doing so, you can evaluate how you're going to use the next 24 hours. You can also do this at the end of the day to evaluate how you spent your day in order to determine what you would or wouldn't want to repeat.

Remember, exercise is a great time filler. The time you spend moving is always a worthy investment toward your good health. The rewards are endless. A short amount of time spent on exercise can transform your physical and mental health. Before you know it, your disposition is on point.

I challenge you to spend some "productive" time on your health. Try it and see!

Body Acclimation
Day 92

It's undoubtedly beautiful this time of year, and with prettier weather people are drawn outside to enjoy this New Year warmth. After a cold winter it feels so good to sit out in the sun and allow your bones to thaw in the early Spring sun. But, there is a truth that needs to be considered. Whatever your favorite season is, your body must acclimate to a new normal temperature. In other words, your mind may be ready to go but your body may respond exactly the opposite.

How does your body respond to this seasonal change? You may feel very sluggish and tired. What is the answer to overcoming this physical reaction? Time – it takes our bodies approximately 30 days to acclimate to new seasonal temperatures. If you exercise regularly, this physical response should be considered as you go forward with your weekly exercise routine. We all should proceed with caution, listening with extra care to the ways our bodies are responding.

Another time to consider body acclimation is when you travel and exercise. Exercising on vacation in a different climate or altitude can be a challenge. Your body doesn't have the time to acclimate, so it's wise to use discretion while exercising in these situations. You may want to consider working out with less intensity before you begin your workout to avoid the possible side effects.

As Spring is upon us now, I encourage you to take it slow for a few workouts. Have confidence that your body will soon adjust and you'll be glad you pushed through listening to your body every step of the way. Our fitness journey is full of mountaintops (extraordinary days) and valleys (hard days), but by golly, we WILL carry on. Onward is the only successful answer.

In and Out of Season
Day 93

The impending change of season is upon us. The lull of winter will soon be behind us, and the certainty of change is just around the corner. Each new season brings about a different result from the one before.

Embarking on an exercise program is much the same. When you begin, you may be very excited and immediately experience great results: lose weight, sleep better, tone up, etc. This is much like the arrival of springtime.

As time goes on, you may slow up some or you may stop exercising altogether. As a consequence, your results diminish, maybe putting you in a season of winter.

Here is an in and out of season testimony:

"Being a very outdoors person, who loves walking and water sports, I started seeing that I was slowing down and thinking it was just age. I really didn't think I would be able to get back to an 'I can do it' feeling." (Out of season)

"For the last two months I haven't been able to work out, and that old slow person has come back and I don't like it. I was able to restart my fitness goals with help and encouragement and the power from within; I realized that I could do it and that 'feel good' person started to come out again." (In season)

Whether you're in season or out of season, remember nothing is impossible. You're either in season or out of season, but let's go forward not basing anything on feelings.

We can all appreciate the benefits and newness a new season brings. There are tough days ahead, too; just hang in there. This too shall pass. There is always sunshine on the horizon and a new energy to be discovered. Stay engaged in your fitness.

It's in the Water
Day 94

I attended a continuing education class this weekend. I love learning, because we can never learn enough. Actually, I rise up daily, ears open and heart ready, to discover something new. So, needless to say, a continuing education weekend is especially exciting when you learn something new about a subject you love.

Water is vital. We will talk about water and it's many facets throughout the year. This learning weekend shed some light on an area that I've never thought of before. We all know that holding water (fluid) weight in our body isn't good. One fact about water is when you drink water your body actually rids itself of excess fluid. Studies have proven water (fluid) has a tendency to be retained; that affects a woman's problem areas.

Sounds crazy, doesn't it? As women age, one common area of weight gain is their triceps area. There have been particular studies that have shown this is a result of the lymph nodes holding toxins and acids that the liver was unable to process due to an overabundance of toxins. By drinking water, you can flush these toxins out of your lymph nodes, resulting in smaller triceps. Wow, who ever knew drinking water can make your triceps smaller? Sounds like a woman's dream come true!

Water is a must for everyone seeking better health and wellness. Ladies in particular, this should give you even more motivation to drink up.

With warmer weather approaching, I challenge you (man or woman) today to be sure to keep water around at all times. If you're thirsty, that's an indicator of dehydration. Make it a point to drink more often than you think you need to so you remain adequately hydrated. It's amazing how simply adding water can set you up for better health.

Got Pain?
Day 95

We've all experienced pain once in our life. When exercising and pain occurs, it's always an indicator of a problem. A lot of my clients say, "I'll just push through." That's not always true. Pain must be assessed. Pain should never be ignored. Do you back off or push through?

The question is, how do you know when to stop or continue?

First, let's address when you need to stop:

When you experience pain that persists. Pain that occurs before, during, and at the end of a workout is in need of medical attention. If you don't listen to your body and continue to push through, it will get worse. Please see your physician.

Secondly, let's address when to continue:

Mild pain associated with normal stress on the body by the demands of exercise will soon diminish. Any type of workout can amplify soreness and stiffness in the beginning but soon goes away about ten minutes into your routine.

Lastly, there is pain from a strain or sprain (acute injury) that needs immediate attention:

As your personal trainer, I am allowed to recommend the proper treatment for an acute injury. Rest the muscle, add ice, compress by wrapping with a bandage, and elevate it above your heart for proper blood flow. Your body is designed to heal itself, but you must give it adequate rest to do so.

If there's any question about your pain, I strongly encourage you to consult your physician. Living in pain is miserable. Your body is amazing and won't lie. Listen to its cues and back off when it tells you to.

Got pain? Listen and obey. You've been given one body, so use wisdom in caring for yourself.

Does Exercise Keep me from Sickness?
Day 96

An apple a day keeps the doctor away. What we eat is extremely important. Does exercise keep sickness away, too? Yes, it does. Exercise boosts the body's immune system. Exercise increases the amount of immune cells that are released into our bloodstream.

Daily exercise has a cumulative effect that keeps the immune system ready and alert. The job of immune cells are to track down foreign invaders, so when these foreign cells circulate at a higher rate than normal, the body is better able to destroy viruses. Exercising regularly is like getting your own booster shot.

I know this to be the truth. Over the past 30 plus years of a committed lifestyle of exercise, I can count on one hand the times I've been sick. I've observed there are not a lot of people in the fitness environment getting sick regularly.

The people who are more likely to get sick usually don't exercise regularly and have unhealthy habits due to not having a proper outlet to handle their stress. Another genre is the elderly; their risk of getting sick increases. The good news is exercise can counteract the sickness that these sectors of people experience.

Exercising regularly can keep a simple winter cold away. Also, in the workplace, people who exercise five or more days a week have reduced their number of sick days. This is one of the reasons why corporations are taking wellbeing more seriously.

I challenge you to faithfully pursue your weekly fitness routine. Discover for yourself how much healthier you've become. This alone should be a big motivator. It's like survival of the fittest. No one wants to be sick.

Digestion is a Pathway to Health
Day 97

I'm going to get a little personal today. I'm going to talk about the bathroom. I'd like to share this because your "potty time" is so IMPORTANT and needs attention.

First thing about "potty time" I'd like to discuss is if you're NOT going on a daily basis. How many times a day do you "go?" Everyone's different. A healthy range is typically 1-3 times a day, but it can vary from day to day. "Potty time" is moving waste out of the body so you can properly remove toxins.

If your "potty time" isn't healthy, your digestive tract isn't either. It may be moving too slowly or too fast. This can lead to an increased risk of chronic inflammatory conditions. The quality of your "potty time" is like the quality of your car engine. It's a direct indication of how well your digestive tract is functioning.

How easy is it for you to "go?" It's normal in our culture to take a phone to the bathroom and spend thirty minutes. The reality is, however, a healthy "potty time" should only take a few minutes, and it should be easy. Straining typically leads to hemorrhoids which are uncomfortable and all too common today. Normal "potty time" is a balance between not having to push or strain and not having so much urgency you can barely hold it.

Digestion is a big part of how we absorb calories and metabolize our food. If things get backed up, everything slows down. You want everything running smoothly. Your goal is to have your digestive tract working properly and efficiently like it's supposed to.

Who would have ever thought your "potty time" was so important? I challenge you to make sure your digestion is on a pathway to health.

Victory is Won One Step at a Time
Day 98

rest day

We've all been discouraged one time or another. We all want to succeed. I've discovered through helping others and in my own journey, it's all about the small steps. Lasting success comes by taking one small step at a time.

The first small step begins with the right mindset, an "I can do this" way of thinking as you approach new ways. Simply saying you'll move for ten minutes daily can reduce anxiety about whether you're doing it "right" or doing "enough." It can keep your "I can do this" mindset positive and accomplish-able. If it's too complicated and your new goals require too much of your time, you will probably lose your positive mindset and quit.

Soon after making small changes to improve your health, you'll find yourself encouraged, desiring to do more. This is when you take the next small step. It's time to implement support.

When you have a specific, easy goal, it's so important to have powerful motivators that remind you to make your healthy choices. You may have moments when you're not excited about your goals, so reinforcements of fitness friends around you will keep you driven to succeed.

Victory is won by knowing that weight loss takes time. You want it to take time because you're making lasting changes while learning a new lifestyle. I tell my clients a quick weight loss is a quick weight gain and vice versa. Your body fights to stay at the certain weight that it's used to. If you weigh 140, it will fight to stay there.

Be confident each time you follow through with a small step. You're making changes that are going to last. Victory is won one step at a time.

Dreams Really Do Come True
Day 99

What's in your closet? Do you have clothes you one day hope to get into again? Have you moved them from room to room or house to house in anticipation to lose the weight to wear that "hot outfit" one more time?

Here is a testimony from one of my clients who never gave up on her dreams:

"We all have those "skinny clothes" in the back of our closets that we just can't get rid of, even if we are 3 sizes too big for them. Well that WAS me! I had clothes that I transferred from house to house I couldn't fit into; just hoping one day I would. In August we were asked to join a company workout class. I figured once a week won't hurt me, so I did it. This once per week class encouraged me to work out more than just once per week.

I joined a gym close to home, and with the help and information provided by our trainer it was easy to know what to do when I got there. I now workout 4-5 times per week. I use things I learn in class to do at the gym. Just the other day a man stopped and asked, "Where did you learn that?" and I told him. A few minutes later I caught him doing the same exercise.

I have dropped "my numbers" tremendously. I've won 3rd place in the company contest. Now I am passing those closet "skinny clothes" on to others and buying new clothes in even smaller sizes. It is a GREAT feeling. It takes hard work and dedication, but with encouragement it makes it easier to want to exercise!"

I challenge you to believe in yourself; your dreams can come true.

Can Exercise Trigger Emotions?
Day 100

Just the other day, I was talking to an awesome client of mine.

We were discussing how exercising seems to stir up an emotional response. Some people might feel angry, joyful, or sad while exercising. Others may even cry, being tears of joy or sadness … whatever the case, emotions are stirred.

Exercise can stimulate neurotransmitter activity in the brain, which may lead to increased emotional intensity. As neurotransmitters like dopamine, serotonin, and norepinephrine increase or decrease in our brains, we may be more aware of positive emotions like enthusiasm, joy, and euphoria (the well-known 'runner's high'). Our bodies can hold tension and negative emotions that can be released during physical activity, too.

Remember the T.V. show *The Biggest Loser*? I would faithfully sit down and watch it every week with notebook and pen, eager to take notes on the particular exercises the trainers would do. But by the end of the show, I was always more touched by the many emotions of the participants than any exercise they did.

I learned that a big part of their weight loss and transformation was allowing the emotions to be released through the exercise process. To conclude, the chemical responses that exercise produces in our brains do amplify our emotions. This response is good and a healthy release.

During your next workout, if you feel yourself getting emotional, remember it's a normal, healthy response. It's good to know that you can walk away from every workout leaving behind unwanted emotions. Or, on the flip side, after a workout you can amplify the good emotions of happiness, sense of accomplishment, and relief.

Each workout always brings something good!! I encourage you to welcome all emotions exercise may bring. It's always worth the sweat of tears and joy.

Does Targeted Training Work?
Day 101

 Boy oh boy, I wish I could say "yes" to this one, but unfortunately the answer is "no." Targeted fat loss, also known as "spot reduction," is a popular idea partly because it appeals to our intuition. It seems perfectly reasonable to assume that the fat you burn while exercising comes from the area around the muscles you are using. Right? Wrong.

There are a few basic reasons why targeted fat loss does not work.

The first reason is that the fat contained in fat cells exists in a form known as triglycerides. Muscle cells, however, cannot directly use triglycerides as fuel; it would be analogous to trying to run a car on crude oil.

The second reason is that many of the exercises commonly associated with spot reduction do not actually burn that many calories, and if you are not burning enough calories, you are not going to lose much fat from anywhere in your body.

Fat loss does not come down to targeted exercises but to the basic principle of how many calories you expend versus how many you take in.

The answer to your problem areas is combining cardiovascular exercises with weight training and sensible nutrition. With those 3 in play, your fat cells will not stand a chance. You can certainly tone up the muscles in your problem areas and it will help a lot as far as improving them.

You must remember the real payoff will come through a committed, intense weekly routine of burning calories and watching what you eat. Then one ordinary day, you wake up and your fat loss has peeled away the covering over those areas and reveals what you've worked for underneath. It's the ORDINARY DAYS of doing what is right that brings about the EXTRAORDINARY DIFFERENCES.

Basic Fitness 101
Day 102

Basic Fitness 101 is a grounding force in this crazy, ever-changing world. When life gets seemingly out of control, we resort back to the basics of life. My faith, family, fitness, and friends are my grounding source. Let's focus on the fitness aspect and how it grounds me and hopefully helps you.

I fell in love with fitness during my senior year in high school. As far back as elementary school, I was always extremely strong and athletic, but I developed some strange eating habits alongside fitness. Food and exercise have been my tools of coping through life's difficulties. I could write a complete book about my eating struggles, but for now let's stick to fitness.

Here are some steps that I consider basic for keeping myself grounded:

Exercise most days. I can personally testify that exercise has kept me sane and productive through all that life has thrown my way. Exercise will be a vessel to help you be an overcomer.

Don't change things up. If you're a runner…RUN. If you're a boxer… BOX. If you're a golfer…GOLF. If you're a biker…BIKE. Whatever gets you going, do it.

Mental psyche: Exercise not only grounds me at my age physically, but also mentally. In my younger days, there was nothing better than an amazing workout and watching my body respond for an upcoming competition. Now, much later in life, every single workout offers a much needed mental release.

Personal Note: When I sit down and write week after week, it has brought healing to my past, made me push through extreme insecurity, and given me an opportunity to help with great understanding and compassion. So, I want to say a BIG, BIG "THANK YOU!" I'm honored to walk with you and am determined to win together.

How to Lift Weights Effectively
Day 103

Have you ever wondered how to fully benefit from lifting weights without hurting yourself? My first experience with weightlifting was in a gym in the 80's. There were very few ladies lifting weights back in the day. A gym atmosphere can be extremely intimidating. My heart's desire is to help you establish a routine that's simple and effective.

Let's apply the F. I. T. acronym to resistance training. These particular steps will give you an effective workout.

Frequent strength training for healthy adults is to train two to three times per week. If you're an older adult or have been sedentary, start with two times per week. Choose light intensity exercises. Spread your resistance training sessions out throughout the week. Rest is key with lifting weights. A forty-eight hour break between sessions is a must.

Intensity strength training is also necessary to grow in your journey and it challenges you. Start with light weights and increase the resistance as you become stronger. The most important key with intensity is to learn the proper technique for each exercise. Do not use momentum or make jerky motions to move a weight. Do not hold your breath. Exhale during the exertion of the movement and inhale during the effortless phase.

Time involved with strength training is around thirty minutes. You should train two muscle groups at a time. Let's use chest and triceps for example. You can do two different exercises for the chest and two different for the triceps, four exercises, repeating (reps) eight to fifteen times each different exercise for five rounds. Time will vary based on each individual.

A weightlifting class or a personal trainer can help you put an effective workout together. Lifting weights will transform your journey.

Salt and Sugar
Day 104

Too much salt is bad. Too much sugar is bad. Too much of anything is bad. My sister sat outside of a health food store one day, called me on the phone, and said, "This store isn't our answer for weight loss." She stated that the people going to the health food store weren't what she expected them to be.

Even at health food stores, with good, nutritious foods available, you can still be at risk for eating too much of a good thing. Let's talk about sugar and salt, adding some knowledge to our healthy lifestyle.

Sugar is everywhere. As we seek out healthy food choices, let's not forget to keep our eyes open to how much sugar our bodies should consume. The recommended amount is no more than 9 teaspoons daily for men, while women shouldn't have more than 6 teaspoons. This amounts to a maximum of 37.5 grams of sugar (or 150 calories) from sugar for men, and 25 grams of sugar (or 100 calories) from sugar for women.

Sodium is everywhere. The recommended daily allowance should be less than 2,300 milligrams. On average, Americans consume close to 3,400 milligrams of sodium per day. Just 1 teaspoon of table salt has 2,325 milligrams of sodium.

Why are sugar and salt considered two evils? Answer: they are both easily overdone in just one meal. Second, not being aware of your sugar and salt consumption can cause some serious health problems.

Consuming too much sugar and sodium can raise blood pressure, which is a risk factor for stroke. High blood pressure can also be a contributing factor in heart disease, kidney disease, and congestive heart failure.

Simply be aware of your sugar and salt intake. Food is to be enjoyed. We all have a God-given conscience. USE IT.

Staying on Track
Day 105

rest day

Staying on track is a key component to any health and wellness success. It's easy to let your guard down, and before you know it the old unhealthy ways of doing life creep back in. If you've found yourself off guard ... there is HOPE.

The mind is a powerful force. Most of us think really negatively of ourselves. If we don't take those thoughts seriously, it becomes extra hard to get our guard back in place. Starting small is a great way to get your momentum back.

Begin your small step by choosing a physical activity. For instance, pull out those exercise shoes and take a small walk. Don't worry about how long or far you go. Ride your bike; a leisurely ride has benefits for your body and mind. Work outside; gardening and yard work are great ways to add activity.

Take the stairs. Even if this is the only thing you do all day, you'll feel stronger for it. You can trick yourself into play. What kids call "play," we often call "exercise." Play a sport, a game, or use the playground equipment to bring the fun back into fitness.

Revive your nutrition. Stir some new excitement; go shopping in a new healthy grocery store you may not normally go to. New ideas about food, or even finding a new health food, can change your mindset and get you back on track.

If you've found your guard down, you're not alone. We've all gotten off track. As long as you get back up after a fall you will eventually outstep your steps backward. Every time you rise up and get back on track, you stay ahead of the game. I encourage you to dust off your knees, get your guard up, and don't look back.

The Man Plan (For the ladies, too)
Day 106

Men, is it possible you're overtraining? The answer is yes. Everyday life activities plus your "training" regime can result in a fatigued body with overuse injuries. But never fear, because I have a suggested plan and it's right here.

Spring is here. These warmer months require a lot more for the men (or the ladies) in the house. Mowing the lawn, home repairs (not to mention the home improvement list that's probably never-ending), and even your golf buddies calling your name, usually mean you're going to be outside a lot more.

My mission is to make sure you stay healthy and strong so you can do it all. So here is the plan. In order for you to stay healthy and active for many years to come, it is imperative that you continue to keep your core strong. Believe it or not, you'll want to keep your resistance training weights light during these warmer months. Each of these exercise elements will help ensure you stay up and about and not down and out.

Developing your core can help to maintain mobility, flexibility, and strength, all of which are critical elements strengthened in the gym, needed around the yard, and appreciated on the golf course.

Lift too heavy too often and you may find when you call on your body to help you mow the lawn, golf, shoot hoops, hike with your son, play volleyball, etc., you end up with an overuse injury.

I challenge you to go light in the gym. Focus on your core strength and you'll be strong and ready for action. You'll be sure to enjoy your hobbies for many long years.

Do Dietary Supplements Really Work?
Day 107

Dietary supplements can help, but they don't perform miracles.

If you're considering taking a particular supplement, I would consult your physician. You should talk to your doctor because dietary supplements are treated more like "special foods." They are NOT regulated by the Food and Drug Administration (FDA), like a prescribed medicine from your doctor.

Dietary supplements can be helpful when you're making choices to begin an exercise program or a new way of eating. Reaching your athletic goals takes a lot of hard work and sometimes a specific supplement can catapult you.

Let's discuss a few fitness related supplements:

Using caffeine for endurance. Caffeine is a controversial stimulant. I purposely drink my coffee about 30 minutes before my workouts because it improves my intensity and endurance. Too much caffeine can cause headaches, irritability, stomach upset, dehydration, and trouble sleeping.

For the guys, Creatine Monohydrate for intensity. Your body makes creatine naturally, and your muscles use it to do high-intensity exercise. A Creatine Monohydrate supplement can boost the amount your body has to work with.

Branch Chain Amino Acids (BCAA). These amino acids are the building blocks of protein. The branched chain types are the three amino acids that muscles can use for energy. Athletes take them after workouts as tablets, gels, or drink powders to spur muscle growth.

Whey protein. Like branched chain amino acids, many athletes take whey protein, usually in a protein shake, after workouts to try to curb muscle damage and boost growth. Most protein shakes have BCAA's in them, so if your goal is simply better health, a whey shake alone will suffice.

I challenge you to always do your homework. There may be a perfect dietary supplement for you. A health and wellness lifestyle is far from boring. There is always something to learn.

Doing Our Small Part
Day 108

All we have to do is get up and move. That's it. All healthy adults aged 18–65 should participate in moderate intensity aerobic physical activity for a minimum of 30 minutes, five days per week, or vigorous intensity aerobic activity for a minimum of 20 minutes, three days per week.

Every adult should perform activities that maintain or increase muscular strength and endurance for a minimum of two days per week. You do NOT need a traditional gym for your muscular strength. Cleaning the house, doing floor exercises with your baby, or mowing the lawn can all build muscular strength.

Our only part is movement. The problem is we want to control the outcome of our results. What we don't realize is we're unable to change our genetics; it's literally impossible. If you really think about it, we have little to do with certain outcomes in life. We must simply do our part and accept the things we can't change.

I challenge you to do something small but powerful. Walk. I challenge you to walk 1-3 miles, five days a week, for one month. There are so many options: to name a few, you can walk outside, inside the mall, around the pool, or around your child's ball practice track.

After completing the challenge, notice your results. Maybe you can take measurements around your chest, hips, and thighs before and after your month of walking. Or put on a pair of tight jeans today and at the end of the month put them on again to see your results.

Doing your small part goes a long, long way. What do you say? Take the challenge with me. There's never a dull moment when we're doing our "small" part.

Nothing Tastes Better Than Being Fit Feels
Day 109

You have made a decision to incorporate exercise into your life. Now you have to prioritize and reorganize your life to include this exercise. You'll soon realize though nothing tastes better than being fit feels as feeling good physically begins to take precedents over bad food choices. I constantly struggle to eat more than I should. Yet, I know if I go back for more food, I won't feel as good.

Being fit looks different for everyone based on individual goals. Thus, we have to make our own choices for fitness. Below are a few suggestions to help you meet your goals.

• Exercising and eating one bowl of cereal tastes good and is satisfying but eating a second bowl of cereal will leave you feeling lethargic and bloated.

• Eating two little pieces of chocolate and taking a walk on your lunch break feels better than eating twenty pieces of chocolate. You'll feel a sugar rush afterwards, but you'll be in a loll thirty minutes later and have to sluggishly finish your work as the rest of the day creeps by slowly. Your body will appreciate the two chocolates and the brisk walk at lunch, and as a bonus, you'll be more alert and energized to enjoy after-work activities.

• Eating one plate of food followed by physical activity tastes better than eating two plates of food followed by hours of lying on the couch watching TV. I choose to exercise in the morning to keep me from falling into the trap of skipping it after work. It is always wise to know your weaknesses.

I encourage you to go after your fitness potential. You will feel better, have more energy, and agree that nothing tastes better than being fit feels.

Find Where You Thrive
Day 110

Having struggled with poor eating habits, I've viewed food improperly. I've looked to food to heal my hurts and satisfy my longings. It always failed me, until I got into fitness. I saw food as something that can give a body muscle mass or fat. Lean meats provide proteins that build and repair muscle. Brown rice is a carb that gives you energy. Even still, I never looked at food as something to be enjoyed.

My love/hate affair with food has been quite a journey. When my children were small, I learned the importance of food presentation. My husband, at the time, would laugh at meals I prepared for my girls. He taught me the key to getting children to eat was in the way I presented it. I had to make it look exciting.

Grocery stores have figured this out. They sell dinosaur chicken nuggets and gummy bear vitamins to appeal to children. I'll never forget a story I was told about starving children. They were served the same food over and over. Eventually, they stopped eating because of the presentation, despite their hunger. They didn't continue to thrive because they needed variety even when faced with starvation.

It's the same with fitness; we must enjoy the variety of health and wellness options and find where we thrive. I had the honor of keeping in touch with most of my clients through the pandemic, and it was interesting to me - some did NOT thrive working from home and others did. Some have experienced great success in their fitness lives, while others have not so much.

Environments and motivating factors help us exist and thrive. Making a change or switching up the presentation stirs excitement. If you're thriving, learn why you're thriving and stay in that particular vein.

Roadblocks for the Aging Exerciser
Day 111

rest day

While driving your car, you've seen road signs that say "detour ahead." Next, you do the obvious - take the detour. I'd like to share some roadblocks and detours for you as you age throughout this journey.

People in their 20's have optimal health at their fingertips. What's the roadblock? Health is usually taken for granted. The detour: establish good habits of exercising on a regular basis.

People in their 30's still have full potential for optimal health. Roadblock? The number 30 gets people down mentally. Detour: simply keep exercise and healthy eating a part of everyday life.

People in their 40's come to the conclusion that there's still a lot of life left. Many people make life-changing decisions in their 40's to get up and do something about their health. Roadblock? Hormonal changes. Detour: seek a physician's guidance to help you get regulated plus utilize diet plans and fitness routines.

People in their 50's don't take their health for granted. Roadblock? Menopause or a mid-life crisis. Detour: continue doing what you learned in your 40's - make regular preventive visits to the doctor.

People in their 60's have either cultivated a strong fitness foundation or they haven't. People in their 60's who've exercised through the years are placed in a league of their own. They typically don't look their age. Roadblock? Flexibility. Detour: Incorporate a stretching program to enhance muscular growth and mobility.

People in their 70's are still in need of a daily commitment of exercise and healthy eating. Roadblock? Recovery time. Detour: It takes a little more time for the exerciser in their 70's to recover.

I challenge you to take the necessary detours to enjoy a quality, healthy, mobile, independent life.

What to Eat Before a Workout
Day 112

Anyone who makes fitness a priority has experienced that moment when a slight tummy growl comes along as you're heading to the gym. The question is, do you grab a snack? Yes. How much of a snack? The calorie amount is important. If you don't address the calorie amount, you could run the risk of eating too much and skipping the workout all together.

Your best bet is a low-fat snack, about 100 to 300 calories, that gives you a mix of protein and complex carbohydrates. The carbs give you fuel to perform a GOOD workout. If you're pumping iron, protein is essential for your muscles. I'd suggest a 350-calorie snack for ladies and probably a bit more for men.

Make sure to eat a little something rather than skipping a snack. The snack will ward off stomach cramps and can reboot your energy levels just enough, so you'll have the energy needed to get in a GOOD workout.

Here are some good healthy suggestions for pre-workout snacks:

- Oatmeal with cinnamon and blueberries or dried cranberries
- Whole wheat toast topped with nut butter and sliced bananas
- Fruit smoothie with yogurt
- Greek yogurt with low-fat granola
- Half of a turkey sandwich
- Raw veggies with hummus
- Whole-grain crackers with low-fat cheese
- Cottage cheese and sliced apples or bananas
- Trail mix with nuts and dried fruit

I would avoid foods that are high in fat or fiber. The digestive process of fats and fiber mixed with a workout can upset your stomach. It takes longer to digest; therefore, it takes longer to deliver energy, and they may leave you feeling sluggish.

I encourage you to gain as much knowledge as you can. When you discover that perfect snack and calorie amount, it's like finding a hidden treasure.

Who Are You Listening To?
Day 113

Are you making much headway in your wellness pursuit? Who are you listening to in this pursuit of positive change? We all have a small circle of support. It's yourself, your circle of friends who become your cheerleaders, and the surprising group of naysayers who are slightly unnerved by this new passion you've embraced. It now becomes a choice of who you listen to.

In this pursuit of fitness, a lot changes because transformation is bound to happen when you make different choices. As a result of your desire for a healthier life, your priorities change, your schedules change, and the people around you may even change. Any change, be it good or bad, causes a disturbance.

Your new change can even stir fear in those closest to you, because they may be afraid you're going to leave them behind. Surprisingly, they can even turn out to be your greatest critics. Oddly enough, they mean no harm, but little do they know their words and actions could be detrimental to your success.

This is the reason to frequently revisit the question, "Who are you listening to?" You must decide to listen to your heart and become aware of those who may be trying to derail you by attempting you to go back to the old you.

Listen to your heart and those who support you and cheer you on in a better, healthier lifestyle. You don't want to forfeit all of your hard work only to make your discontent friends content. Instead, you can encourage them to join your journey, and in turn they may thank you. I challenge you to ask yourself who you're listening to.

How Can I Get Nice Abs?
Day 114

We all share a common desire for nice abs. How can you get nice abs? The answer is: abs are made in the kitchen based on the 80/20 rule. This rule of thumb is 80 percent nutrition, 20 percent exercise. If you aren't seeing progress, you may want to take a look at your weekly menu. Diet is a small word with endless options.

In order to sculpt a flat, toned stomach, you need to do two things: burn fat and build muscle. Having low body fat equals more muscle definition. You can religiously exercise (which is your 20%), but your six-pack won't be visible if it's hiding beneath layers of fat that can only be changed through diet.

A good place to start in changing up your diet is to eat healthy fats and lean proteins. When my daughter was 14 and starting to become very aware of her body, having constant questions, I would say, "Fat doesn't make you fat. It's the excessive amounts of carbohydrates that lead to extra weight."

I have requests all the time to do core/abs work, and that's great. To maximize the payoff from those core workouts, I'd suggest incorporating some particular foods that are known as "belly-slimming foods" into your diet, such as eggs, chicken breast, fish, and lean cuts of beef.

My goal is to leave you with these simple facts that may point you in the right direction to help target your waistline. I realize everyone is different. What may work for one person may not work for the next. I encourage you to start trying new things with your diet. Changing up your eighty percent will guarantee a difference in your abs. You'll never regret trying new things, but you WILL regret never trying.

Regular Exercise Produces Self Confidence
Day 115

If you exercise regularly, you're accomplishing mini goals that lead to a more confident you. I'm not talking about a puffed up muscle head that can't take his eyes off himself in the mirror. If you've ever seen that, it's most likely a big telltale sign of insecurity and placing value in the outward appearance, not the gratification of accomplishment.

What is confidence? Confidence is having trustworthiness or reliability in a person or thing. It's believing that person or thing has the ability to succeed. Confidence is different than arrogance, which are often times confused as the same. Arrogance is offensive. If you've ever been around someone that's arrogant, you can immediately feel their display of superiority, self importance, or overbearing pride.

Why is having confidence so important? When you're on a quest of bettering yourself through a constant pursuit of better health, it bleeds over into every aspect of your life. Your work performance, relationships, and quality of life improves. When you're healthy, your confidence will make difficult situations easier to handle.

As you seek good nutrition and complete a walk, run, or exercise class, know there's more inside you to be birthed and developed. A newfound determination is birthed, and before you know it, you'll have larger borders and fewer limits on yourself.

Remember, it's never too late to begin. Don't limit your goals and desires. Be determined to stretch yourself. Run your personal race with confidence. Who ever knew that exercise is a link for success? Try it and see; you'll be a more confident you – guaranteed.

Felt Like Giving Up Lately?
Day 116

Have you felt like giving up lately? Spring's here, and you may be reading this a couple of pounds heavier. Or maybe you just haven't lost the weight you thought you would have by now. Those New Year goals are long gone. Now here you are, still the same as you were when you first started, left with extra frustration. Whatever state you find yourself in, be persistent and don't give up.

One of my clients was in this very state. She was very frustrated with her fitness plan. Week after week she came to class, but the weight wasn't coming off as she hoped. She was considering just giving up. After a little discussion, we made a small tweak in her diet and *voilá*, the weight started coming off. She experienced the breakthrough she had been working so hard to achieve.

You too can make small changes, whether it be in your fitness routine or your diet. The golden rule here is not to give in or give up. If you make small changes and stay consistent, your perseverance will pay off with the results you're after.

You must remember the results may not show today, they may not even show tomorrow, but hang on until you physically see the pay off. Regardless of the time frame, I challenge you to keep pressing forward and don't give up. Your victory is inevitable.

Why Does Your Weight Fluctuate?
Day 117

Did you know when you step on the scale, you're not just measuring muscle and fat? That number represents the combined weight of your bones, organs, and bodily fluids. So, go ahead and expect your weight to slide up and down on the scale....IT'S NORMAL.

We must stay encouraged that a higher number on the scale may have NOTHING to do with your health and wellness progress.

Here are some variables as to why you may see a bump up on the scale.

Water. Water is attracted to sodium like a magnet, so when you eat a lot of sodium, you're more than likely hanging on to extra water.

The potty. I know it's not the most comfortable thing to talk about, but this can affect the scale in a big way. It's most healthy to eliminate waste daily. If you don't, this can cause you to weigh more until your body releases the waste it's hanging onto.

Carbohydrates. Your body has a huge capacity to store carbs. Did you know your body has the capacity to store at least 500 grams? One slice of bread equals 15 grams of carbs. When you eat more carbohydrates than your body immediately needs, you WILL store the leftovers. They hang around until they're needed for fuel.

Fat. To gain one pound of body fat, you have to eat 3,500 more calories than you burn. For example if you eat 500 more calories than your body burns every day for seven days straight, you'll probably gain a pound of real fat weight.

If you've experienced your scale increasing by one pound or so, no worries. Regroup ... get up ... dust off and get back in the game. Weigh out all the factors. Whether your scale goes up or down, simply keep moving forward.

Go Green Fitness
Day 118

rest day When sunny, warm days begin to come around, the gym can sometimes look a little dull, dreary, and boring. When this happens to you, take your fitness plan "green." Throw open the doors and go outside for your workout, enjoying the fresh air. There is healing to be had in the freshness of the new spring air.

Here are a few good "green" fitness alternatives to the gym:

- Do my workout video outside. That's my favorite place to work out.
- Find the nearest walking/running trail.
- Do water aerobics.
- Challenge yourself while riding a bike: keep your abs in tight; find hills to ride up, or stand up while riding.
- Do walking lunges up and down your driveway.
- Do some push ups on your porch.
- Use your steps for triceps, dips, or uneven squats.

The freshness of a new season is to be experienced. Get creative. Go outside and go green. Don't miss out.

Is Juicing for Me?
Day 119

rest
day   Juicing seems to be here to stay. Juicing has been heralded as nearly miraculous for just about everything from losing weight to preventing cancer. Because of this, the juicing trend has spread fast.

Lots of moderately health-conscious people frequent juicing establishments daily/weekly. For others it has become a way of life; they even juice at home. Today, I'd like to talk to the novice person who might want to try juicing and experience something healthy and new.

The definition of juicing is extracting the natural fluid, fluid content, or liquid part that can be obtained from a plant or one of its parts, especially from its fruit. One of the first things to keep in mind is juicing has calories. Juicing is a great way to get those vitamins and minerals you may not otherwise get if you're not a vegetable/fruit eating kind of person. But still, you must consider that you're drinking calories. It's always good to be conscious of your overall caloric intake.

Fruit is key in making all vegetable juicing more palatable. The kinds of fruit you should use in your ingredients are any kind of fruits ending in berries (e.g. strawberries, blueberries, blackberries, raspberries, etc.). These particular fruits have a lot of antioxidants.

Seeds are a good ingredient to consider using. Seeds are super antioxidants for our bodies. Some examples are flax, chai, hemp, and wheatgrass seeds.

Above are a few basic tips for trying something new. I encourage the avid juicer to share your knowledge with others. In our health and wellness journey, we must always stay open to new things. New things are what keep your body responsive.

Good health is achieved from putting vegetables and fruit in your body. I challenge you to try a juice drink today.

Crossroad Decisions
Day 120

If you're seeking better health, let me encourage you by shining some light on the word 'crossroad.' The definition of crossroad is "a place where roads intersect; a point at which a vital decision must be made." A fitness crossroad is becoming aware of seemingly insignificant choices and decisions that can lead you to continued improved health.

Life is all about choices and decisions. The choices most people are aware of are the big ones, such as the school you choose to attend, the home or car you buy, or perhaps the biggest one, the person you marry. However, each small choice and decision can be as equally important as becoming aware of things.

I heard a really great sermon on "Choices and Decisions." The gist was this: you're where you are right now in life because of one CHOICE or DECISION you've made. The same is true for your health. Where you are physically right now is a direct result of your accumulated choices and decisions. You might weigh heavier than you'd like or be thinner than you'd like, or you might have once had better muscle tone and stamina.

The hardest one is finding yourself in unforeseen circumstances, beyond your control. This happenstance can bring on new stress. These demands need your undivided attention, which takes energy from the smaller, better health choices. However, you need to remember that this is temporary and get back on track as soon as you can.

Take heart; simply being aware is golden. It will always keep you heading in the right direction.

Fiber and Fitness
Day 121

You usually don't hear about better fitness and fiber in the same sentence, but today I'd like to connect the two. To have any success in your personal fitness, it first takes having a healthy heart. Without a heart, we'd all be doomed and there would be no fitness plan without one.

First, it's good to know women need 25 grams and men need 38 grams of fiber per day. Most Americans don't get the adequate daily recommended allowance. The average adult only eats 15 grams of dietary fiber per day. Do you know how much fiber you consume?

I'd like to challenge you to find out how much fiber you are personally consuming. If you discover you need more fiber, please make sure you drink more water. As we know, fiber helps with digestion, but without water all you'll get is a stopped up digestive track.

Adding fiber to your diet will help the most important muscle in the body, the heart.

The benefits of fiber to heart health are:

*Lower LDL ("bad") cholesterol levels

*Lower blood sugar levels in people with diabetes

*Lower blood pressure in people with high blood pressure

*Lower risk of heart disease

*Lower risk of diabetes

*Healthier weight and lower rates of obesity

Adding fiber can assist in weight loss, too. Foods that are high in fiber tend to be lower in calories. Some top sources of fiber are: beans (all kinds), cornmeal, bran, raspberries, blackberries, prunes, dark leafy greens, broccoli, okra, cauliflower, sweet potatoes, carrots, and pumpkin.

We mustn't forget fiber is beneficial for better fitness. It's exciting to know this journey is never ending and there are always new (and old) ways that can stir up and spark better fitness.

Don't Let the Scales Weigh You Down
Day 122

What's your number? When you step on the scales and the number is higher than you expect, how do you handle it? Does it kick you into extreme discipline, or do you find yourself hopelessly rummaging through the kitchen cabinets eating everything you can lay your hands on? Or are you good with your number? If you are, then be on guard and aware of thoughts that may say "you deserve a break today."

From as early as Junior High School I can remember stepping on the scale and it saying 140 pounds. My girlfriends weighed 120 pounds. The misunderstanding of a number that is ideal for me led me down a road of eating disorders. My weight made me feel shameful. My guilt lay so heavy on my shoulders that it would drive me into the kitchen, grabbing whatever food was in sight. Or I would get a wild hair and lose weight, followed by rewarding myself with mounds and mounds of food, which has been a destructive cycle of mine for more years than I can remember.

I encourage you to not get fixated on a number. I challenge you to find peace where you are today. Don't cast your highs and lows on what the scales say or on how someone else looks. Refrain from hanging your fitness hat on a number.

Gauge your success on how your clothes fit and everything you have accomplished. Before you jump on those scales to check your weight, I say WAIT. The days of my youth have taught me a valuable lesson. I step on the scales once a year when I go get my physical. If you're not sure how you're going to respond to the results, then put the scales away.

Remember, You Can Do Fitness…Believe It!

Rest or Sleep
Day 123

Did you know that rest and sleep are vital components of fitness success? They both serve important benefits to the body. The problem is, these two components are often overlooked and pushed aside. Not only are they beneficial but also serve two different purposes.

Rest is needed for recovery. Everyone has a different rest schedule and amount of recuperation that is needed for their individual success. This can only be determined by the individual. No one formula will work for everyone, because our bodies differ. The amount of rest one needs is dependent upon age, gender, weight, and fitness level.

For example: An older individual that begins a weekly workout regimen will need a lot more rest than a young competitive bodybuilder. A good tell-tale sign that your body is in need of rest (no matter what age, gender, weight, or fitness level) is a sore muscle or overall body fatigue. You should never feel sore or tired at the beginning of a workout. A sore muscle or overall body fatigue is your body's way of communicating that it needs rest.

Sleep is needed for muscle growth. You don't build muscle in the weight room. Actually, you're tearing down muscle fibers as you weight train. Muscle growth takes place when we're sleeping. The growth hormone, HGH, is released while we sleep. This is why sleeping is so important. HGH levels increase during deep sleep, which often begins 30 to 45 minutes after falling asleep.

We must use wisdom in knowing when our bodies need rest or a good night's sleep, or both. We all have a common desire to be the best that we can be. You're worth the time and effort it takes to provide the best care for yourself … that includes rest and sleep, too.

Body Pain
Day 124

There are two kinds of body pain: good pain and bad pain. There is nothing worse than experiencing bad pain! It makes you grumpy, miserable, and on a hunt for relief! On the other hand, there's a good body pain. Good pain gives you a sense of accomplishment that makes you come back for more.

Everyone hurts to some degree during exercise. We've all heard the saying, "No pain, no gain." The truth is some pain is the price you pay for working out and improving performance. However, it's crucial to distinguish between types of pain. Good pain is the type of pain that is attributed to the muscle strengthening process. Bad pain is the kind of pain that is associated with injury.

Good pain is experienced after a workout, which produces stiff and sore muscles up to 48 hours after exercise. This comes with the territory, especially when you're trying to improve your fitness performance. You might feel great during the workout, but the next day you may find it tough to climb a short flight of stairs.

Bad pain is experienced when pain doesn't go away after your warm up. Exercise doesn't involve excruciating pain. Stop immediately. The more you work out and ignore bad pain, the more you place yourself at risk for serious injury.

Good and bad pain can be alleviated by the RICE method (rest, ice, compression, and elevation). If this particular pain persists, it's considered a chronic pain. If you're experiencing any type of pain for longer than a week, it's best to consult your doctor. Now that you know a little more about pain, don't let mild soreness stop you from exercising. On the other hand, don't ignore pain that persists. See your doctor. Right pain is right gain. Know the difference.

Fat is the Question
Day 125

Gyms usually have a display of fat to share with potential new members to motivate them to join. If you've never seen this display, it's a yellowish, rippled mass about the size of a tenderloin. This vision makes anyone want to lose weight, but believe it or not, this display can be misleading.

Did you know there are two kinds of fat? There's a good and bad fat. The bad one is called "white fat" and the good one is called "brown fat."

Everyone is born with white fat. It's the predominant form of fat in the body originating from connective tissue. We make white fat bad when we consume more calories than we can expend because the body stores fat when food is abused. America's overeating and sedentary lifestyles should make us all cautious of developing white fat.

Everyone is also born with brown fat. It's reddish-brown in color and packed full of power producers which give the cells energy by turning calories into heat. Babies have an abundance of it. It helps keep them warm as they exit the womb.

You can't see brown fat by just looking at your body. For the most part, it's sprinkled in between areas of white body fat. You can generate more brown fat by exercising. Exercising outdoors in the wintertime can promote more brown fat and so does getting enough high-quality sleep.

These facts should motivate us to make healthy, moderate eating choices and to exercise regularly. A healthy lifestyle can minimize white fat and generate brown fat. That is a most encouraging bonus!

Joint Safety
Day 126

rest day We all know exercise is good for everyone. It's good for your heart, helps with weight loss, and provides a variety of health-related benefits. But, at the same time, exercise comes with a certain degree of injury risk, and depending on the activity, it can also put a lot of stress on your joints.

For some, this might be a good excuse to say, "Well, there you go; I don't need to exercise." Or some may ask, "How can I avoid the risk of injury and not place too much stress on my joints?" The key is to exercise safely and to choose activities and movements that reduce your risk of injury, pain, or other complications. There are a lot of different solutions, but today I'd like to share some safety tips that would apply to almost everyone.

Wearing the proper footwear is an investment. But, good footwear for your specific activity can prevent injury and pain, as well as the expense from doctor's visits and physical therapy.

Exercising with proper technique. It's easy to fall into incorrect alignment. Unless you know how to correct yourself, it would be a good idea to hire a qualified instructor. A qualified fitness professional can point out basic safety in your particular workouts.

Warm-up stretching. A warmup safely prepares the body for the increased demands of exercise by generating heat, increasing circulation to the muscles and joints, and lubricating the joints for activity.

Cool down stretching. The cool down brings your heart rate back to normal slowly and safely, which helps prevent pooling of the blood in the extremities. This helps maintain and increase joint mobility.

I challenge you to take precautionary measures that reduce your risk of injury by practicing joint safety.

Adaptability
Day 127

As I was exercising the other morning, I started to think about the word, "adaptability." So I looked it up in the dictionary after my workout and found that it meant to change so as to fit a new or specific use or situation. I've been in the fitness industry since 1985. The one thing I know to be true is you must be adaptable to thrive and survive in your personal health and wellness walk.

I'd like to share my personal journey with adaptability. Each decade of my life has looked very different. In my twenties, my workouts were as hardcore as I could make them, and I had no body aches or pain. My thirties were baby-making years, and though my life changed forever, fitness was still a consistent part of my daily life.

In my early forties, I started feeling minor aches and pains. I adjusted my workouts accordingly, and it was no big deal. Then in my late forties, I began making accommodations to manage more serious aches and pains. In my mid-fifties, I faced surgery, and after two total hip replacements and the pain and therapy that went with them, I still worked out. Now, in my late fifties, I've become a high-maintenance exerciser, modifying most of my exercises to suit my needs and abilities.

Our bodies will change, and we must find a way to accept the changes that are taking place. Once we do, we can better assess our health and fitness and properly modify our regimen accordingly.

I challenge you to be adaptable with your exercise. Don't be afraid to adapt accordingly as you feel your body changing. With proper care and management, your body can stay fit and strong the rest of your life.

Can Music Help My Workout?
Day 128

Who would have ever thought that the music you listen to during your exercise time can help your athletic performance? It's true. Preferred music can give you a performance edge just like workout supplements can. Today we're going to talk about how music can affect your workouts.

There is a term called "arousal regulation," which means music can act as a stimulus. Music can take the place of a workout supplement or stimulant and help athletic performance. Music can be used prior to competition or training as a stimulant, or it can be used as a sedative to calm anxious feelings.

To "psych up," most athletes use loud, upbeat music that is usually played in a gym setting for best athletic performance. Or softer selections can help to "psych down," usually played in yoga classes for best results. All in all, music provides arousal regulation that encourages an optimal mindset.

Everybody who has experienced exercise has experienced the "good pain" that exercise creates. Playing music that you enjoy during a workout can actually divert you from that "good pain." It's called dissociation.

During exercise, music can narrow attention, diverting the mind from sensations of fatigue. This diversionary technique, known to psychologists as dissociation, lowers perceptions of effort.

Effective dissociation can promote a positive mood state, turning the attention away from pain. More specifically, positive aspects of mood such as vigor and happiness become heightened.

Music can impact and positively improve motor skills. Think back to elementary school days and your physical education lessons, which were usually set to music. Music accompanied dance, and play created opportunities to explore different planes of motion and improve coordination.

I challenge you at your next workout to enjoy the music, have fun, and train hard all at the same time. Music brings great rewards.

Emotion Commotion
Day 129

What is the first emotion that you felt this morning when your feet hit the floor? Maybe it was happiness, anxiety, dread, or loneliness? Unruly emotions can sneak up on you during any occasion, but they don't have to overtake you.

Each day, it's important that you quickly recognize what emotion you are dealing with. If it's a nasty one, you should then ask yourself if you are going to get it under control or if you are going to allow it to stomp on you and steal your valuable (never to be seen again) day? In other words, who's in charge - you or some emotion that you have given control to?

Many a day I've used exercise to help derail a potential emotional train wreck that could have overtaken me only to ruin my day. Here are some examples when exercise has served as a positive outlet for every single emotional state I've encountered. It's helped me by soothing my anxiety, been a great stress release, and enhanced a sense of euphoria through chemical releases, which left me happy and far from depression.

Exercise can't stop the unwanted emotions from coming. They're just a part of life. However, when exercise is a part of your life, you have a wonderful way of dealing with the tough days.

Remember you're in charge of you. Use exercise to your advantage in all areas of your life. You now have the perfect physical antidote for dealing with unruly emotions - EXERCISE.

Cardiovascular Training 101
Day 130

Looking at the foundation of any successful fitness plan, you must have all 3 key components: diet, strength, and cardiovascular training. We discussed strength training first because I'm a musclehead at heart.

Speaking of heart … everyone living and thriving has to have a working heart. So obviously your heart is your most important muscle. Did you know your heart is a muscle? Your heart is a muscle just like any other muscle in your body. In order for it to become strong, it must be worked just like your other muscles.

Cardiovascular training is what works the heart muscle. So, if you fail to fit cardiovascular training into your weekly routine, it will weaken over time. The danger of a weakened heart muscle can be the cause of a variety of negative health effects, like high blood pressure, thyroid disease, kidney disease, or diabetes.

We can't neglect our #1 muscle … we all need our hearts. The good news is it's never too late to get your heart muscle stronger. Exercising your heart will keep it in shape and healthy. This is accomplished by putting a demand on your heart through continuous movement for at least 20 minutes most days, like brisk walking, running, biking, or any activity that requires continuous movement for longer than 20 minutes. This continuous movement is defined as cardiovascular (aerobic) activity.

Not only will aerobic activity strengthen your heart, it will also increase your metabolism. An increased metabolism means an easier time maintaining your weight, losing weight, or even gaining a healthy weight.

Cardiovascular training shouldn't be an option. Let's make a decision to NOT neglect the heart. We can't live without our hearts. I challenge you to get out there and find some cardiovascular training that best suits your individual needs.

A Win-Win
Day 131

Setting goals keeps the spice in a health and wellness journey. Goals keep the bar raised to constantly challenge you to the next level. Most of us have no trouble setting a goal. It's the process after the goal has been set that is difficult.

Today, I'd like to talk about the process of achieving your goals and help you with some win-win strategies and some thoughts to steer clear of.

Win-win when you create a plan. Steer clear of waiting for "someday" to roll around.

Win-win by starting small. Steer clear of focusing on too many things at once. Try focusing on one goal at a time.

Win-win by writing your goals down. Steer clear of not giving yourself a deadline. A little pressure to get things done is a good thing.

Win-win when you're specific. Steer clear of absolutes. Avoid the words 'some' and 'more,' as in "I will get SOME exercise" or "I will eat MORE veggies." Believe it or not, this way of thinking leaves too much wiggle room to bail out.

Win-win when you leave room for failure. Steer clear of expecting perfection. Persistence is key. Accept the fact that you might not make it on the first try.

Win-win when you track your progress. Steer clear of fooling yourself into failure. Memory can be pretty selective, especially when you're making progress. You must remember the biggest discourager can be yourself.

Win-win by rewarding your success. Steer clear of beating yourself up over failure. Negative thoughts are usually in our heads, telling us what we're doing wrong every day. Take time to recognize your progression.

Goal setting rocks. Sure the in-between part is grueling, but it's so worth it in the end. Simply TAKE ACTION. You won't regret it!

Full Potential
Day 132

Here are a couple of questions frequently asked of fitness trainers: "How do I get the most out of every workout? How do I burn the most calories/fat or gain the most muscle in every workout?"

The best answer I've found is to exercise to your full potential. To exercise to your full potential is to put forth 100% effort in every workout. That 100% is broken down into 90% mental readiness and 10% practical application. We spend a lot of time discussing how to be victorious on the mental side of the fitness battleground; however, we can't ignore the practical application of exercise.

I may have my mind all primed, convinced, and confident I can do it, but then I need to step up and actually do the work. The 10% is needed to see success. The most time-efficient and effective way to get the job done is through both strength and cardiovascular training. My videos address the resistant training segment.

The practical application of exercise added to your day equates to far less than 10% of your full 24-hour day. It simply doesn't take much time. I challenge you to make the choice to practically apply yourself and guarantee in time you'll experience results.

God has designed your frame, nutrition plan, and exercise regimen. Ask Him for it; listen and obey what He has called you to do. Don't be bound to man's teachings and man's rules. Isaiah 55:8, 9 (NIV), "For my thoughts are not your thoughts, neither are your ways my ways," declares the LORD. "As the heavens are higher than the earth, so are my ways higher than your ways and my thoughts than your thoughts."

I encourage you to continue to seek out new things. Learn your full potential.

Sugar or No Sugar
Day 133

rest day Once upon a time, I lived next door to a brilliant woman who later became my best friend. Upon meeting her, I very quickly learned we shared a love for the human body. We were also both interested in helping people grow in health and wellness. She has her PhD. I always told her, "You're too smart for your own good."

After a couple of conversations about my body pain, one afternoon I received a knock at my door. I opened the door, and my new friend boldly proceeded to tell me my pain was caused by wheat and sugar. We laugh when we look back and reminisce about that awkward visitation.

From that day forward, I went on a quest to omit wheat (gluten) from my diet. It gave me tremendous relief, but I told her I would NOT quit sugar. End of story. Sugar was my kryptonite, but I never cared … I loved it. A decade later, I had body pain once again, and without seeking help, I knew exactly what to do. It was time for me to deal with my sugar intake.

Sometimes we don't want to change because change is associated with pain. I'm talking about the pain of breaking a bad habit, but that's good pain, my fitness friends. In order to face my 35 years of addiction, my body pain had to surpass the pain I would experience withdrawing from sugar after having eaten it in very large amounts most of my life.

Health and wellness is not for the weak at heart. You're not meant to do it alone. We need each other. So, let me ask you a question: "Do you eat sugar?" You have your own personal experience. Share your story; you never know who might benefit from it.

146

Staying Fit to Best Help Others
Day 134

I was traveling the friendly skies recently and before take off, heading for the runway, the flight attendants did their standard greeting and safety speech. This time something they always say got my attention. "In case of an emergency and your oxygen masks drop, please place your mask on before you assist others."

Now, if you didn't know better, you might think that seems a bit selfish, but the truth is, we all need to be at our best in order to best help others. Cultivating a consistent time and place to exercise is probably one of the best things we can offer others.

We can get things backwards sometimes. Going to church is a good example. People have told me they need to stop smoking, drinking, or doing whatever habit they have that makes them feel unworthy, before considering going to church.

If you're a church folk like me, you would agree that "anyone is welcome just as they are." I was literally one step away from suicide the first time I saw the inside of a church 24+ years ago. I feel funny sharing this today, because GOD has done such a HUGE miracle of healing in me.

People have expressed to me their desire to start eating better or lose 10 pounds before beginning an exercise regimen. The truth is, you don't have to be fit to get started, you just have to get started to be fit. Did you catch that? You don't have to be fit to get started, you just have to get started to be fit. We can get the simplest things backwards sometimes.

The next time you think twice about starting a fitness journey, don't wait another second; start it. Remember, staying fit is the best way to help others.

Can What You Eat Age You?
Day 135

What you eat can age you. Maybe it hasn't yet, if you're in your 20s or 30s. As you approach your 40-plus years, it matters more about what you eat.

None of us want to age before our time. I'd like to share some basic factors to keep us on track at any age.

Poor-quality foods that are unavoidable: these particular foods consist of processed carbohydrates like pasta, bread, and baked goods. The problem with these foods is that they contain too much sugar and sodium. Facts about these two evils (if abused) can make you look older than you are.

Too much sugar or sodium can lead to eventual damage in your skin's collagen. Collagen is what keeps your skin springy and wrinkle-resistant. I know we're all destined to lose collagen, but let's not speed up the process. Poor-quality foods negatively affect the body due to inflammation. Foods to avoid are potato chips, french fries, doughnuts, and sugary pastries.

Inflammation is not good for your body. If we don't pay attention to inflammation, it can set us up for premature aging. A factor in the aging process is your body being in a chronic inflammatory state. We want to keep sugar and sodium (processed carbohydrates) to a minimum to avoid excessive inflammation.

You can eat foods to help cut down on inflammation. Fruits and vegetables can help eliminate this natural swelling. Fruits and vegetables are good for your skin, too. Look at people around you and their skin. Some people have an extra glow about them. Watch what they eat. I'll bet fruits and vegetables are a big part of their diet.

What you put in your mouth affects what you see in the mirror. I challenge you to eat your fruits and vegetables.

Faithful Fitness
Day 136

When I was exercising the other morning, thinking about fitness (as I love to do), the word "faithfulness" came to mind. I began to think about relationships and fitness. I thought about how we all want loyal, committed relationships in our lives, and fitness is no different.

They both have character traits of faithfulness. How we treat others and how we treat fitness will show in the results we reap. As a child, my momma always said, "Do unto others as you would have them do unto you." We can adopt this phrase to fitness: "Do unto your fitness as you would have it do unto you!" Bodies don't lie; they are an outward display of how we treat them.

How to develop faithfulness fitness like a good relationship:

Remain loyal when the day in and day out mundaneness loses its excitement. Keep exercise top priority. Find new ways of doing the same thing. There are many ways to eat chicken; it gets boring to cook it the same way all the time. Doing squats gets boring, too. Change your normal squat routine; learn new ways to squat. Spicing up your bland rice and pastas is no different than your cardiovascular workout. Atmosphere adds great spice.

Believe in yourself. You must settle this argument deep within. You ARE worthy. You ARE confident. You WILL believe in yourself. You CAN do it! This is not arrogance but a belief that must be established from the beginning. Whether you're overweight, underweight, healthy, unhealthy, we all want to look and feel our best. Results must begin with a belief and vision that you can accomplish your dreams and aspirations.

I finished my morning workout, realizing fitness has been my faithful friend all my life. I encourage you to discover that, too.

Pre-workout Drinks
Day 137

There is a lot of hype about pre-workout drinks. They affect each individual very differently. Oftentimes, with trends like pre-workout drinks, you usually find a gap between fitness and health. A good pre-workout drink could give you an awesome workout but might not be the best choice for your health.

Being conservative when it comes to shooting for optimal health while being your best self, the most important question to ask is, do I need a jolt to get me going for my workout? You must decipher if your body is telling you to take a booster (pre-workout drink) or to take a look at your nutrition, sleep, or relaxation. It's all connected.

Without getting too technical, I do believe that the safest way to see and understand meaningful change in health and wellness and what your body can personally handle is through starting with what's inside. This is done through getting your blood work done regularly. A healthcare provider can help you best understand your individual genetic and physical traits. Then, from your results, you can get a nutritionist consultation for personalized recommendations you can implement.

Some pre-workout formulas are designed to give an almost instant improved appearance to your muscles with an ingredient called Arginine Alpha-ketoglutarate (also known as AAKG). This particular nonessential amino acid has been proven to increase nitric oxide production in the body, which in turn ensures more blood, oxygen, and nutrients are delivered to the muscles.

Caution should be taken in implementing a pre-workout drink for your daily workout regime. The number one reason for this is because the Food and Drug Administration does NOT regulate the safety and sale of nutritional supplements. So, whether you're conservative or not, use wisdom.

Is Gluten Linked to Inflammation?
Day 138

Not long ago, I wrote an article on "the gluten-free diet" being a fad. A doctor recently challenged me to try a gluten-free diet to help with joint inflammation. I was a skeptic but gave it a shot.

I've found in the last couple of years, my knees swell by the end of the day. I thought this was my new norm. About a month into my gluten-free diet (being a skeptic the whole time), I saw that the SWELLING IN MY KNEES WAS GONE.

Gluten is a protein found in grains like wheat, barley, and rye. Gluten gives our favorite foods that special touch. It makes pizza dough stretchy, gives bread its spongy texture, and is used to thicken sauces and soups.

Are you gluten sensitive? Check with your doctor. Gluten intolerance can result in a wide variety of symptoms. Arthritic pain, osteoarthritis, rheumatoid arthritis, and generalized bone and joint pain can be symptoms of a gluten intolerance or sensitivity. Gluten intolerance requires different treatment than just a sensitivity to gluten.

Switching to a gluten-free diet is a huge task. It can be difficult and frustrating to adhere to such a lifestyle change. Creativity and patience will help you find foods to substitute and satisfy your needs. Consulting with a dietitian can be most helpful for tips, recipes, advice, and motivation.

Through my own personal testimony, a gluten-free diet is linked to inflammation pertaining to my particular body. A personal testimony is powerful. It can help others. On our constant quest to find the best nutrition and exercise plan to meet our individual needs, stay open to new ways and ideas. Listen to the testimonies of others. New discoveries may work or may not work for you. We never know unless we try.

It Works!
Day 139

rest day

Today, I'm going to share a truth. If you do it, IT WORKS. I'm going to say something very simple, almost too simple to say, yet profound. Usually, people seek better health and wellness for a ONE-TIME event, expecting quick results, only to quit after the ONE-TIME event is over. You must stay ready year-round and open for any opportunity that might present itself.

Below are examples of one-time events that need year-round attention:

- I want to look great in my bathing suit this summer.
- I'm getting married. I want to look stunning in my dress or tux.
- I'm single again; I want to get in shape.
- I'm going to my class reunion.
- I'm in the wedding…OH MY!
- I want to fit back into my pre-Covid jeans.

The answers to all these events is (of course) to go to the gym, hire a registered dietitian, and hire a personal trainer. Do what needs to be done and don't stop. Move forward and maintain so you don't regain. Keep the habit and don't quit.

This may sound cliche, but this is the answer and it works. It works if you move your body most days. This means 150 minutes of moderate to intense aerobic activity every week. Also, practice resistance training that works all major muscle groups 2 or more days a week, and BINGO … you've got a lifestyle.

Keeping fitness a big part of your life, all year long, makes you ready for any event that may come your way. Then, when that ONE EVENT is here and gone, and all is said and done, I encourage you to continue exercising. You'll continually be ready for the biggest event of all, called LIFE. Keep up the hard work…IT WORKS.

What NOT to Eat
Day 140

rest day What is a good, healthy diet? "Lean proteins, vegetables, and fruits" - no matter what literature you read on the subject of diet, you'll find these three food groups. Why? Because they're rich in nutrients and supply what your body needs to thrive and achieve optimum health.

Today, let's talk about foods that need to be avoided. This is important because eighty percent of wellness success comes from what you eat. Avoiding certain foods or even minimizing one or two things can produce some BIG results.

Have you ever heard the term "keep it simple sweetheart?" This is a good rule of thumb to live by when making food choices that can be difficult and confusing. So let's discuss two food groups that can be avoided that provide virtually no health benefits.

White bread and refined flours generally provide zero nutrients. They've been virtually stripped of all vitamins, minerals, fiber, and other important nutrients. Refined white flour has also been bleached with chlorine and brominated with bromide, two chemicals that have been linked to thyroid and organ damage.

Diet anything. Many so-called "diet" products on the market today have many additives. Diet products contain added chemical flavoring agents to take the place of fat and other natural components that have been removed to artificially reduce calorie content. Instead, stick with "whole foods" that are as close to nature as possible. This includes high-fat foods grown the way nature intended. Your body will respond surprisingly well.

Simple changes within these two food groups can transform a life. Diets need to constantly be changed because our bodies are in constant change. It's a very rewarding feeling to discover what foods your body responds to best and what foods it doesn't respond to at all.

What We DO Have
Day 141

Human beings have a tendency to focus on what's lacking in their lives and at the same time miss out on personal successes. You must make a conscious effort daily to focus on what you do have and fight against thoughts of lack. This pertains to health and wellness in a big way. Ask anyone around you if they're satisfied with the way they look physically.

Let's be determined not to be consumed by unsatisfactory thoughts that ruin everyday freedoms.

Examples of the wrong focus and the truth of right focus:

Example 1: Body Image. Most of us are unhappy with our height, physique, or appearance. It's connected to a perceived inferiority. The root issue stems from a cultural preference or societal norm that fosters negative thinking about your attractiveness.

What you do have: Learned self-acceptance. You can't change your face or your height; but you can work out to sculpt a better you. Make sure you're making decisions that make you happy and healthy, not because you feel pressure to look a certain way.

Example 2: Performance anxiety. Comparison and perfection hold us captive to the wrong values. First of all, we usually compare ourselves to the wrong thing. We live in a world that's great at measuring and comparing externals.

What you do have: How do you combat comparison and perfection? Celebrate who you are. There are many wonderful things about your life. You have much to celebrate. You're entirely unique.

Let's be determined to keep our focus on what we DO have and steer ourselves away from what we don't have. We're only on this earth for a short time; let's embrace all things with great celebration.

It's OK to Skip a Workout
Day 142

There are times when we have valid reasons for skipping workouts. You shouldn't beat yourself up for missing a day or even a week of workouts if you have legitimate reasons to skip.

I hope these justifiable reasons to miss workouts help ease any guilt you may carry:

You're crazy busy. If you're too busy, you're too busy. I speak grace to you today.

You're injured. Your ultimate goal is to give your injury the essential time to heal. If you don't rest, continued pounding to the injured area is putting more strain on your injury. If you ignore rest, you run the risk of chronic pain or surgery. Talk to your doctor or physical therapist to find out what activities you can do with your injury.

You're recuperating from surgery. In the case of a major surgery, or even a minor one, the last thing your body needs is to work out too soon. Your body is already working overtime recovering; let your body heal.

You are experiencing lack of sleep. Sleep is as important as your actual workouts. Your body is healing as you sleep. Chronically skipping sleep to exercise brings on fatigue and even injury.

You're sick. If your illness is above the neck (for example, a runny nose or sore throat), you can safely work out (unless you have a fever). If your illness is below the neck (for example, stomach problems, lungs, or full-body aches), it's best to rest.

You just completed a major athletic event. If you ran a 1/2 marathon, full marathon, or an all-night race, you're entitled to a day off from your usual workout. Allow yourself to recover properly.

Don't feel guilty another second for skipping a workout when you have a good reason to do so.

Raw Passion
Day 143

Passion is defined as a strong like or desire for or devotion to some activity or object, or something for which you have a deep interest. We all have some level of passion or deep interest regarding how we look or how we feel, but what else?

What else strikes a chord with you? In addition to how you look or feel, where else does your passion lie? Is it to live longer? Avoid having a heart attack? Seeing your children grow up and marry? Hike the Appalachian Trail? Cycle cross country? No passion is too small or insignificant, nor is there one that is too great.

Let whatever desire that lies within you be the driving force to seek a life of health and wellness. Maybe you, or someone you know, is very passionate about a particular issue in life. We all possess some degree of passion. In pursuit of that passion, you must be in good health to be your best. I want to assure you it's never too late to take action toward your desire that's been pushed aside because you thought it was an impossibility.

Summon your level of passion to rise up and get going. It only takes a seed of passion to produce a harvest of success in your health and wellness. If you haven't discovered or acknowledged what you're passionate about, I encourage you to do so. Plant your seed and water it today. The "water" for your seeds is taking action. Water ignites the growing process for your seed.

Take action; exercise with me today. Take a brisk walk outside, or engage in a fitness activity. Recognize your passion and take action to make it grow. I challenge you to plant, water, and harvest; you'll never regret it.

It's Worth the Wait
Day 144

If you're in this battle of health and wellness to win, you must brace yourself for the long haul. You can look at your exercise days like a must do, with no ifs, ands, or buts, because it's now a part of your life. Pumping iron may seem as silly as snowboarding in a swimsuit. Even riding your bike might feel like it's a waste of time, believing you aren't getting any results, but that's a lie, lie, lie.

You might become shortsighted and think, "What the heck! I'll have double cheeseburgers most nights and forget about those lean meats and fresh vegetables." Before you do … think, think, think again. Your newfound lifestyle is making a difference. It's a matter of grabbing hold of the simple fact that it's making differences toward your betterment.

Make sure you're believing the truth. Keep exercise in your weekly routine, because the harvest of goodness is coming. I encourage you to continue reaching for something healthy again and again. Always be open to trying something new, because you'll soon discover it does matter. You can do this.

Keep your exercise clothes handy. Pack an extra outfit in your car for an unforeseen opportunity to say yes to exercise. Your daily workout schedule should be just as important as your next planned meal. Treat both as a priority.

It'll be worth the wait; one ordinary day, boom, the results you've worked so hard for are here. Your pants will be loose, the scale is 5-10 pounds lighter, or you simply feel better because of healthier dinner choices.

You'll pack your exercise clothes with excitement now, because you finally see those benefits. REMEMBER THE BATTLE IS WON BECAUSE YOU DIDN'T QUIT THE FIGHT. Have a healthy and active day. It's worth the wait.

Wants or Needs?
Day 145

Most of the time when someone has a desire to become fit, it's for an upcoming occasion. Very rarely do people come to the gym because of a need expressed by a doctor warning them of a high risk for diabetes, high blood pressure, high cholesterol, or another health problem stemming from an inactive lifestyle.

Let's decipher the differences between wants and needs of health and wellness.

NEEDS of health and wellness:

• Maintaining a healthy weight: Without any physical activity in your life, you'll be prone to gain weight. Most sedentary adults between the ages of 18 and 49 gain one or two pounds each year.

• Mobility: Flexibility exercises such as stretching and yoga help enhance our range of motion, prevent injury, and reduce pain and stiffness. Even if you have limited mobility, you can still benefit from flexibility exercises to prevent or delay further muscle atrophy.

• Energy: Persistent fatigue is on the rise. Physical activity combats feelings of fatigue and low energy.

WANTS of health and wellness:

• A nice body: We want to achieve our image of a nice body whether it includes nice muscle tone or six-pack abs.

• An upcoming event: Reaching for short-term goals to attend a special event only provides short-term results. I encourage people to seek a permanent, healthy lifestyle.

• Revenge body: Unfortunately, we all care what certain "someones" think of us at various points in our lives. This can motivate us to lose weight just to prove something.

Our primary focus should be our NEEDS of health and wellness, and in turn, our WANTS will manifest in one way or another. So, what do you say? Let's push forward so we can enjoy both the needs and wants of health and wellness.

Grab the Bull by the Horns
Day 146

rest
day
Today I want to tell you about a client who has traveled down the weight loss road before, but until last year had never included exercise in the equation. Even as her workload increases, her commitment to exercise never decreases. Week after week she makes the decision to keep pushing on. Her diligence has produced astounding life changing results.

Here is her story:

"In February, I decided to get myself back to a 'healthy' standpoint and hopefully feel better and have more energy. Well, at this point (Dec 09), I have lost almost 60 pounds and 8 sizes in clothes! I really do have more energy and feel great!

Last spring our company had a 'contest on improving your numbers' (HDL, LDL, Cholesterol, etc.). From February 09 to June 09, mine dropped to acceptable ranges for all except my BMI, which improved 6 points but needed to be more to be considered acceptable.

In addition to all this great news, I won the contest and $300. The $300 was great but not as great as how I feel. My goal is to hit the ground running after the holidays and drop the other weight I want to lose. I want to work on maintaining this for the rest of my life."

Obviously exercise is a VERY important tool in body toning, weight loss, and in maintaining for the future. While a healthy weight is certainly something to strive for, it doesn't always have to be our main focus.

Exercise has made her feel great. Everything else achieved is a bonus. Without a doubt, exercise and consistency are the essential tools to achieving life changing results. I challenge you to diligently work on your fitness just as my client did and let exercise work for you. You'll love the benefits.

You Are Here
Day 147

"You are Here." This phrase is often seen on a map located on a kiosk at the mall, Disney World, and other places. By referring to them, we can find where we are and where we want to go. Then, we can plot our course and travel in the direction of our destination. Sure, we may check our GPS gadgets along the way to see precisely where we are located in comparison to our desired destination. Yet, the bottom line is this: how we get there doesn't affect our ultimate arrival.

Achieving our fitness goals is no different. We must get a fitness plan (a map) in play to begin our journey. The biggie for all of us setting out to make a difference in our fitness level is assessing where we are today. Just like a map or GPS says, "You are here," a daily assessment of our individualized plan is needed to keep us on track and moving forward toward our goals (destination). Then we must stir up encouragement along the way by referring to our map each day with determination to move forward no matter what obstacles arise.

Below are some simple examples of what to put on your map. These are simple items you can check off to keep you feeling victorious and motivated to move forward.

- Drink your water quota
- Get at least ten minutes of cardio most days
- Plan to do one day of resistance training each week
- Practice good posture
- Push a little harder
- Try something new
- Do a recovery workout

In conclusion, by accepting yourself where you are at the beginning, you'll have less frustration along the way and better enjoy your journey. You are here; now do something to get one step closer to your destination.

Outdoor Fitness
Day 148

Summer is approaching, which means schedules will change. Kids get out of school; family vacations are planned, or some good ole family get-togethers will be in store. Between work and summer family fun, a routine trip to the gym can be tough.

The good news is the days are longer and warmer, which makes walking, jogging, biking, and swimming great ways for getting in a cardiovascular workout! That doesn't mean you still can't do a good muscle-building workout, too. You've just got to be a little more creative with your outdoor exercise regimen.

Here are some simple strength-training exercises to incorporate with your outdoor workouts to get the ultimate benefit for your time without having to go to a gym for muscle building.

1. Push-ups. This is a power movement that will keep your chest, shoulders, and triceps toned.

2. Pull-up. This is also an upper-body power movement. Pull-ups target the upper back, biceps, and shoulders. This exercise isn't as easy to do as push-ups due to requiring access to a pull-up bar.

3. Dips. This particular exercise targets triceps. In order to successfully accomplish this exercise, you'll need a chair or bench.

4. Jump squats. This is considered a lower-body power movement. It's great for all the muscles in the lower body (calves, quads, hamstrings, hips) and core.

5. Side drop lunges. This is another lower-body power movement that is great for abductors, adductors, hamstrings, and glutes. You'll need stairs or a curb for this exercise. Stand sideways about 2 feet from the stairs or curb, hands on hips. Lunge sideways onto stair/curb then repeat with other leg.

6. Planks: this core movement tightens and tones your abdominals.

7. Being fit this time of year is a blessing!! Happy outdoor fitness!

Where is Your Focus?
Day 149

It's easy to quit something when things get uncomfortable, challenging, or inconvenient. The truth is, however, that it's the hard things in life that render the best results. Exercising is good for you but so many times we simply drop out of the game of fitness simply because we lose focus.

Your life's focus will change as you're on this earth longer. What we deem as important may not be so ten years from now. So one sure way to stay encouraged is to focus on what you do have and not what you don't have.

Below is a list of unhealthy focuses in the area of health and wellness.

• You want to be skinny or look a certain way. There's nothing wrong with wanting to look your best and better yourself, but your focus must be on allowing your body to respond the way it needs to whether that be through muscle tone or weight loss.

• You beat yourself up for not getting results or not getting them fast enough. There is nothing wrong with wanting to achieve results, but you can't place a time frame on a forever task. Health and wellness isn't a part time gig, it's a forever thing—a lifestyle for a lifetime.

• You compare yourself to others. This focus will make you crash and burn very quickly. It's okay to become inspired by others but to compare yourself to others will lead to giving up, depression, or anxiety. A proper perspective is to focus on your own achievements and make goals from your last accomplishments.

Where is your focus? I challenge you to dig deep and find the right focus. Surround yourselves with people who share the right focus, and cheer each other on in this race of a lifetime.

Who Said the Race is Over?
Day 150

Most of us hit the floor running each morning—racing through our days trying to accomplish everything we consider important. In the hustle and bustle of your daily life, it's important to consider exercise is just as consequential. As you contemplate each new day, new week, and new opportunity, I encourage you to make good choices regarding your health and wellness. Time has a way of getting away from us and before we know it a year has gone by.

Whether we like it or not, life itself is movement. So, therefore, we might as well jump in with it to create the atmosphere we desire. Let's join in the forward motion and take action. Let's be determined to stay with the race forward while there is life in our bones and air in our lungs.

Below are some strategies for keeping in the race.

- Begin your day with exercise. It's a great jump start.
- Sit outside and eat lunch. You'll be amazed at what fresh air can do for your mind and body.
- Eat a healthy lunch (Whole foods are my personal favorite).
- Walk after work or go to the gym before going home.
- Be creative with your movement.

Remember to make choices that help you finish strong. There are so many healthy choices to discover. When you seek betterment, you can be confident you gave it all you've got! Don't stop being creative. Seize every exercise and wellness moment. When the day is drawing near to a close and I haven't reached my calorie goal, I march around the house with two incredible dogs. Make it fun. Don't let anybody tell you, including yourself, that movement can't be accomplished. I'm here to tell you the race ain't over.

Push Forward
Day 151

As this year has progressed, I'm sure you have discovered a new normal surfacing whether you like it or not. You may have new regrets from yesterday or a challenging new hope for tomorrow. You may be facing new problems in such areas as weight gain and out-of-control eating. These new problems might leave you with new fears, overwhelming anxiety, and isolating shame. With all this uncertainty of life, it's more important than ever to find a healthy outlet for stress.

You must identify these "new" problems and deal with them in constructive ways. If you don't, your health and wellness will be greatly affected.

Here are some simple ways to be physically constructive.

• Hit something. Learn how to play tennis, golf, table tennis, volleyball, etc. Get boxing gloves and hit a punching bag.

• Work out to your favorite music. You can create the perfect playlist or lyrics that match how you feel and then head to the gym or your designated workout area. Even if you don't feel motivated to exercise by music, it can still make the time go by quicker and even refresh your soul.

• Take a dance or dance fitness class. There are many live and online classes you can try. Try them all to discover which one you like best. Shake your booty, have fun, and dance your body to better health. Free yourself from the adverse effects of stress.

• Let it go. Problems occur when we don't pack up our tents after we've dealt with our issues. The longer we dwell in them, the more they affect our physical health.

Whatever you're facing, it may be time to deal with it, but do NOT forget you mustn't stay there. Push forward. Don't be left behind.

Am I Making Progress?
Day 152

If you've been working really hard for the past six months, but you feel as though you've got nothing to show for your efforts, don't quit. If you feel discouraged because you've tried everything under the sun, don't retreat. Don't give up. I'd like to share some things that might help expedite your progress. Before you allow yourself to think one more discouraging thought, let's take a look at your lifestyle and ask these progress questions.

Question #1: Am I eating too much? Sometimes, you might think you've done good by making all healthy food choices, but the problem is, it's easy to exceed your caloric intake beyond your caloric expenditure for the day.

Question #2: Am I eating enough? On the flip side, you could be putting yourself through unnecessary misery by eating an amount that feels like enough but it's really not. Believe it or not, under eating almost has the same effects on your body as if you overeat. Your body needs calories. It needs fuel to function. If you're not providing yourself with an adequate amount of protein, carbohydrates, and fats, then your body will find ways to store them.

Question #3: Am I stressed out? Stress produces a hormone called Cortisol. When your brain is telling your body it's stressed out, cortisol is released into your body in excess. While some amount of cortisol is necessary to stay alive, chronically high levels will negatively impact fat loss efforts.

If you're eating healthy regularly, you're making progress. If you're doing anything physical, you're making progress. This journey isn't for the faint at heart. You've got to dig your heels in for a lifetime. Your progress is cultivating a quality life.

Can the Scale Keep You in Bondage?
Day 153

rest day Can the scale keep you in bondage? It absolutely can. What you weigh has nothing to do with how you look. With the non-exerciser, weighing is a good starting tool. It can be used to place you on the right track in the beginning. But for the consistent exerciser, it can be a stumbling block.

How many times have you stepped on the scale full of hopeful anticipation, only to be disappointed by the number staring back at you? Suddenly, all the hard work and the great sense of accomplishment you had vanishes. Immediately, you tell yourself, "I've failed." No matter how hard you try, you can't lose weight.

I'm here to tell you that if you're exercising regularly, put away the scale. With each individual body, no one really knows the "scale number" at which you'll look and feel your best. Most people get stuck on a silly scale number to measure health success.

Do you find yourself in bondage to the scale? Do you weigh yourself daily or even multiple times a day? Get rid of your scale. The idea of giving up the scale can be scary. But I guarantee that once you do it, the bondage to it goes away.

Exercise WILL change your physical body inside and out. When you exercise, your body mass index immediately begins to change. Due to the new healthy, physical demand that you're placing on your body, your body's mass is guaranteed to become denser. Density weighs more.

We're all on a journey to be set free from everything that is holding us back. Don't let the scale measure your self-worth or progress. Put the scale away. Break free. Be determined to have a more accurate self-image and better overall relationship with your body. Scale free.

Injury, Injury, and More Injury
Day 154

rest day

Injuries are no respecter of persons. I was sitting watching my daughter's gymnastics class the other night, looking at all the leg boots, arm wraps, knee braces, and ankle braces on all the young athletes. Whether you're young or old, injuries can happen to the best of us. We train as hard as we can, push our bodies to their limits, and those nagging aches and pains always somehow manage to turn into an injury at some point in our fitness journey.

So what do we do? Most of us will probably want to "suck it up, buttercup" or "stick it out" and continue training, but what about the consequences of not letting an injury take the time to heal? A minor injury can turn to chronic pain quickly. Injuries need immediate attention before they take a turn for the worse.

A great way to treat a minor injury is with the R.I.C.E. method.

Rest: Is required. Your body is speaking to you through your pain. It's saying, "lay off!"

Ice: Helps reduce swelling and provides temporary short-term pain relief by reducing blood flow to the injured area.

Compression: Just like ice, compression can help reduce swelling. Getting rid of swelling is important, because when swelling occurs, the injury can take longer to heal.

Elevation: This is another useful tactic to keep swelling in check, and it works best when the injured area is raised above your heart.

This method of rest, ice, compression, and elevation reduces the swelling quickly, alleviates pain, protects the injured area, and accelerates the healing process. Your goal is to elevate because blood and fluids need to flow away from the injury to reduce swelling.

Blah...Belly Fat!
Day 155

Most of us have unwanted belly fat. If we put on a couple of pounds, it always seems to show up on our belly. A big culprit in retaining belly fat is a hormone called "cortisol." As I discussed belly fat with my doctor friend, he told me to emphasize that cortisol is the only cause of belly fat.

Cortisol levels change all throughout the day. Cortisol is one of the first things an emergency room gives a trauma patient. So, cortisol isn't all bad. What is cortisol? It's the primary stress hormone. Your brain's hypothalamus plays an important role in cortisol production. This gland responds to a perceived threat by signaling an alarm to the rest of your body, causing your adrenal glands to release a surge of cortisol. Cortisol provides a sudden burst of energy by increasing the glucose in your bloodstream.

Constant elevations in cortisol can increase your risk of several serious health disorders, including obesity, fat gain around the mid-section, and heart disease. The good news is that regular exercise and other lifestyle changes can play an important role in helping prevent health risks due to an overexposure to cortisol.

During exercise, your body uses cortisol to help metabolize fat for fuel. Regular exercise helps control your cortisol levels and reduces the stress this hormone places on your body. We're all going to experience physical stress at some point in our day, if not each day, and at least once during our week. As we implement a regular, weekly routine of exercise, we can't go wrong.

Next time you get stressed, lower those cortisol levels. I challenge you to get those exercise shoes out and move for 30 minutes. You can now be encouraged that exercising is helping metabolize cortisol for fuel. That is motivating!

Cellulite...Oh My!
Day 156

Cellulite has always baffled me. You can't say a person has cellulite due to being overweight. Thin people can have it. Fit people can have it. Even those who maintain a healthy weight and healthy body fat percentage can have cellulite. The bizarre fact is some unfit and overweight people may not have it at all.

What exactly is it? Cellulite is simply visible subcutaneous (below the skin) fat cells that bulge the skin, giving that particular area a dimpled appearance to the surface of the skin. A common term people use to describe it is "cottage cheese" or an "orange peel." Cellulite can occur anywhere on the body, including the abdomen, arms, and calves.

A fat cell can shrink and can have a diminished appearance, but eliminating fat cells isn't possible. Once a fat cell has been produced within the body you can never get rid of it. Creams, treatments, massage techniques, and other cellulite therapies do NOT get rid of cellulite in a permanent way. They may help the appearance of cellulite as the size of your fat cells decrease.

Cellulite makes us all feel self-conscious. I wish there was a certain exercise to take it all away. It takes a combination of cardio exercises and resistance training to help reduce cellulite by burning fat from all over the body to enhance fat loss.

Having an active lifestyle can keep new fat cells at bay. Exercise is important for not allowing cellulite to accumulate in the first place. God did design a certain amount of cellulite to safeguard our survival. We do need a certain level of body fat. Fat is necessary and healthy for normal body function.

I challenge you to seek being healthy. Overcome your imperfections by determining to live comfortably in your own skin!

Hypertrophy or Atrophy?
Day 157

Human beings must keep their minds and physical bodies stimulated in order to stay on a path of productive growth. Even though our brain is not a muscle, there are parts of our brains and muscles that are stimuli and need action for growth.

The brain is an organ that is made up of neutral tissue needing to be exercised through cognitive functioning like memory and attention. Just like brain matter, muscles have memory that needs to be exercised, too. The skeletal muscle tissue, which is responsible for helping to maintain physical function, includes the ability to walk, climb stairs, get out of a chair, or lift objects.

These are things that determine our independence as we age. Let's discuss what happens if we DO keep muscle building a part of our lives, called hypertrophy, or if we do NOT, which is called atrophy.

Muscle hypertrophy is attained by implementing some sort of weightlifting into part of your weekly routine. When adding a weightlifting routine, you'll be guaranteed that muscle stimulation will produce continued muscle growth. A practical example is lifting groceries.

Muscle atrophy occurs when unused muscles shrink. This can materialize if you're bedridden or unable to move certain body parts due to a medical condition. This is why physical therapy is so important.

Some muscle atrophy is inevitable. As we age, beginning in our 30's, we begin to atrophy by losing volume and muscle mass. If we regularly exercise, we can continue to keep muscle mass even as progressive deterioration happens. We lose as much as 50 percent by the time we are in our 80's or 90's. It's important to exercise as we age.

Your body is important; don't sit and waste another second!! There's good work to do that requires your best health.

Water Functions
Day 158

 Just how important is water? It's VERY important! Whether you exercise or not, water is vital and drinking it can make you healthier.

A person can lose water due to: activity levels (including talking), humidity, and sweat. In general, the female body is made up of 55% water; men, 65%. The human body's blood is comprised of 90% water. When an individual says they don't like water, it may be because they haven't created a habit.

Truthfully, the body craves water and needs it. Here are a few important functions that water plays in the body.

Water in the blood. Water is needed in your blood to transport nutrients and glucose (sugar) to the muscles. Sugar is our energy source. Without glucose we have no energy.

Water in the urine. Keeping your body hydrated eliminates waste products. It acts like a vacuum cleaner, ridding itself of toxins. You'll be cleaner on the inside and have healthier looking skin, too.

Water in sweat. As you hydrate yourself, your body has a better ability to produce the sweat needed to keep the body cool through the skin. If you're dehydrated, you'll have a greater chance of becoming overheated.

Water in saliva. Every time you have a meal or snack, make sure you have a glass of water on hand. Water in your saliva and gastric secretions aids in digestion.

Water throughout the body. Water is needed to lubricate your joints. It acts as a cushion for the body's organs and tissues. If you're hydrated, you may lessen your risk for injury.

Water is vital. If you're not a water drinker, I challenge you to begin with small steps. Start with one glass today. We all have the desire to be the best we can be. Cheers to water!!!

The 80/20 Rule
Day 159

In fitness, health, and wellness, our food choices represent eighty percent of our victory. This hard simple fact shouldn't discourage us. In fact, knowing this truth can truly set us free.

The goal of becoming our optimal best is what we're all working towards. However, all too often this thing called food, the very thing we need for survival, can be the very thing that trips us up and keeps us in defeat.

Instead of defeat, there is victory and freedom to be found in this area. The keys are to keep working at it, continually be open to learning new things, and never giving up. There are resources all around us that can give direction where we may need help. Many examples of resources come to mind.

One example is of a client that found her answers and freedom through Weight Watchers. Another client of mine found answers and freedom when she omitted snacking at night. One more example is a client who began making healthier food replacement choices that brought her answers and freedom.

This big vast area of food can be tackled and conquered simply by staying open to new ways of eating. My biggest heart's desire is for each one of you to find something that works for you and for you to be able to walk in freedom. Too many times I've watched people be consumed, obsessed, and in bondage to how and what they eat. This is no way to live your life.

Sure, the 80/20 rule won't change. I challenge you to be persistent on being free when it comes to your eating. Find what food choices work for you and enjoy your life.

Keep It Going
Day 160

rest day I believe all group workouts should include a good pep-talk. Halfway through a hard workout, I would repeatedly encourage my class to "keep it going." Simple as that may sound, these are three powerful words. They apply both to exercise and life.

We keep it going to complete a hard workout. We keep it going when life gets difficult. Consistency with exercise and life sets us up to win every time. Positive things happen to our bodies when we keep it going and exercise consistently.

Exercise will make us feel happier and help with weight loss. It's also good for our muscles and bones and increases our energy levels. It reduces our risks for chronic disease, helps keep our skin healthy, and improves our mental health and memory.

Reminding ourselves of these simple benefits will help us push through the temporary pain and get us a win-win outcome every time. We may face unrest, toil, hardship, and storms in so doing, but the very things that cause frustration and unease can also produce victory.

We MUST push through adversity and constantly strive for betterment. If we do, we will reap the benefits. We must also count it a blessing to exercise every day because it helps our mental approach to life.

So I challenge you to rise daily and learn to love the benefits gained by pushing through challenges. Rally your strength by giving yourself frequent pep-talks. Stay positive and encouraged and just keep it going!

Did You Say Intensity?
Day 161

rest day Intensity plays a big role in our results, but there's a delicate balance. When you enter a phase of your workout that's intense, you should really be listening to your body's response. Exercising at the correct intensity is crucial, and if ignored, you can invite acute and chronic injuries.

Here's a look at exercise intensity and how to make it work for you:

How you feel is one way to measure exercise intensity. Perceived Exertion is a subjective measure of how intense an activity feels during your performance. It's measured based on the amount of exertion by a scale of one (least amount) to ten (max amount). For example, what feels like a hard workout (nine) to you, can feel like an easy workout to someone else (three).

Your heart rate is another measure of intensity that offers a more objective look at intensity. The higher your heart rate is during physical activity, the higher the exercise intensity. Once you understand your maximum intensity, you can really get creative. When you're doing aerobic activity, such as walking or biking, you can challenge yourself through how your intensity correlates with your elevated heart rate.

Exercise intensity is also reflected in your breathing, your sweat, and how tired your muscles feel. Being aware of all these factors can make a really fun, challenging workout. You can do a combination of moderate and vigorous activity, preferably spread throughout the course of your weekly workouts based on these particular body cues.

Again, reaping the most health benefits from exercise is determined by your exercise intensity, but you must remember the importance of balance.

I hope you'll explore and discover new heights with a new wisdom to keep you in this wonderful game of fitness. It's AWESOME.

Cardio Checkup
Day 162

Cardio exercise has so much to offer. Want a strong heart? Do cardio. Want strong lungs? Do cardio. Want rejuvenated, glowing skin? Do cardio. Want to remove the toxins from your body? Do cardio. If you didn't catch my drift, DO CARDIO.

Here's why - the heart is a muscle, and like all muscles, it must be exercised to get strong. If you are doing cardio that produces a sweat and at least somewhat labored breathing, then you are exercising your heart and lungs. In addition, the sweat you are producing, whether a lot or a little, is not only cooling your body, but it is also pushing out the toxins that are stored within your body and pores. An accumulation of toxins can contribute to disease, infection, and overall bad health. So, needless to say, sweating is good. Another wonderful example is when you do cardio it's like you're stirring up a stagnant pond of muck and flushing it out through your body's personal filtering system, your pores and skin.

Notice I didn't mention fat loss. So often we associate losing fat with doing cardio. While cardio is an important factor in assisting with fat loss, resistance training is the key component here. This particular truth earns a page of its own. Later discussion.

So let's keep moving! It doesn't take much. Just as little as 10 minutes of cardio most days (preferably 20 minutes) can make a difference. Challenge yourself by increasing your intensity levels during your cardio workout this week. You'll soon discover that your heart and lungs are getting stronger. When you wash your face, take note of your skin. Cardio rejuvenates the skin. There may be a brighter face staring you back in the mirror. Watch, expect, and witness your overall wellness improve.

Get Your Motor Running
Day 163

Have you ever thought that during the first few minutes of working out you just might not make it? This is a normal feeling for every single person that begins a workout, no matter what fitness level you fall under. The task of exercise simply feels physically overwhelming. The good news is that feeling only lasts a few minutes.

The first five to ten minutes of working out are always the hardest. During this time your body is warming up. Warming up is essential for preparing your body for more strenuous exercise/activities.

During this brief period of time your body's core and muscle temperatures are increasing. This increase in temperature signals your heart and respiratory rate to also increase. This process of increasing body temperature and oxygen makes the muscles more loose, supple, and pliable, preparing them for more vigorous exercise.

Whatever exercise you choose to do first, be it cardio or resistance, will feel the hardest during those first few minutes. Once you get your motor running, your second wind will kick in and you will feel energized and ready for the intensity of your workout. This will also leave you feeling confident enough to lift heavy weights that felt like concrete before.

Whether you're a beginner or a professional exerciser, remember your body has to have five to ten minutes of warm-up time. So, when the dreaded feelings come, I encourage you to push through. That sluggish overwhelming feeling that happens to us all will pass quickly.

Binge Eating
Day 164

What exactly is binge eating? Binge eating is an uncontrolled ingestion of large quantities of food within a short time period. These episodes are often accompanied by feelings of guilt and hopelessness. We've all overeaten at one time or another, most notably around the holidays or on special occasion. I think we've all gone back for seconds on Thanksgiving, or had an extra slice of cake on a special occasion. So when does the occasional overindulgence cross the line into the realm of real binge eating? It isn't always easy to define.

If your weeks turn into months filled with sessions of overeating followed by guilt, or the lines between enjoying a small piece of pie and eating the whole pie become obscure, it might be an issue of binge eating.

How in the world are we to keep binge eating at bay? The biggest rule of thumb is to eat a balanced meal at every sitting. A balanced meal consists of protein, complex carbs, and a fruit or vegetable. This type of eating keeps your blood sugar levels regulated, and in turn, keeps your body's hunger cues stable so you don't have uncontrollable urges.

Most Americans typically eat too many carbohydrates and little or no protein at each meal. This leaves an individual less satisfied, placing their body's hunger cues out of balance. According to the US Department of Health and Human Services, they recommend two daily servings of three ounces per day of protein. That's a total of six ounces per day. If you divide those six ounces between your three meals, you'll more than likely keep your body regulated.

Remember, even the healthiest eaters aren't perfect. It takes a while to change habits. It's the combination of your choices over time that create an overall healthy lifestyle.

DO IT!
Day 165

 My pastor brought forth an amazing message that correlates very closely with a journey of health and wellness. He said:

"- Don't rehearse it (the bad, negative, impossible, etc.)

- Don't nurse it.

- Disburse it (let go of your thinking of the bad, negative, impossible, etc.)

- And let GOD reverse it (He can make ALL things good, positive, and take our impossibilities and make ALL things possible.)"

This relates to fitness because it's sooooo easy to rehearse why we can't exercise or eat right – nursing all the times we've tried to change, to lose weight, or to simply better ourselves. Therefore, I'm telling you (and me) that it's time to disburse that kind of thinking and allow GOD to light a fire under our tail; get up and do something about where we find ourselves! DO IT!

How do you rehearse it?

*My family needs dinner.   *I'm too tired.

*I've got to run errands.   *My job is TOO much.

Instead rehearse this:

*I'll cook a crockpot dinner so I can exercise today.

*Tired or not, I'm simply showing up.

*I'm going to be time efficient with all responsibilities.

*I'll take a break to eliminate stress so I can be a better employee.

How do you nurse it?

*I'm a fat slob.   *I can't help it.

*My life is terrible and nobody loves me, so I'm going to sit on this couch and sulk.

*What's the point of all that eating right and exercising? I always end right back up in this place.

Instead nurse this:

*I'm NOT going to talk bad about myself.

*I absolutely CAN have self control.

*If you're feeling like life will never get better, STOP!

*Be determined to rise up, walk out your front door, and be a blessing to someone else.

What do you say? DO IT.

Carbohydrates
Day 166

Carbohydrates…it's hard to live with them, but you can't live without them. The human body needs carbohydrates. Where we falter is in the amount of carbohydrates that we eat. The nutritional mainstream is still advocating a large amount of carbohydrates be consumed daily according to the food pyramid. It's too easy to take advantage of the carbohydrate segment of the food pyramid. For this reason I don't fully agree, but we can all agree that carbohydrates are the source of evil when it comes to health issues and obesity.

Bottom line is too many carbohydrates consumed makes us put on unwanted pounds. We've been programmed to think that eating fat is what's making Americans fat. This is simply not true. We are carbohydrate overloaded.

So do we eliminate them altogether? NO. Carbohydrates are essential. They are the body's main source of energy and vitally important to the efficient functioning of many systems. When you consume carbohydrates regularly in your diet, they're providing your body with the energy it needs to maintain necessary processes of growth, metabolism, brain function, and digestion.

A simple way to gauge your daily intake of carbohydrates is to measure YOUR full fist at every meal. This is a great tool to help you maintain portion control and safeguard against too many carbs.

There's not a quick fix for too many carbohydrates. Don't omit carbohydrates thinking this will help you lose weight faster. Omitting carbohydrates from your diet in the short term will hasten weight loss. But if you take this route, your body immediately becomes unbalanced, leaving you with uncontrollable cravings.

We're after a healthy mindset to feed our bodies what is best for the long haul. We have a lifetime to invest in ourselves. Let's invest wisely to be the best we can be.

Exercise Works
Day 167

rest day Today, I'd like to share two simple golden nuggets. What if you don't exercise regularly? If you don't, I challenge you to reconsider because ... it works. Exercise works. Sunday, my pastor preached on faith and patience. We need both "faith and patience" to hold onto until what we are believing for comes to pass. Well, it's the same for exercise.

When you do your workouts, it's in faith. You're expecting all your hard work and sweat to produce results. Right? Right. But your hard work must be mixed with patience. The two golden nuggets are faith and patience. Patience is time, which combined with your faith makes exercise work.

Faith's definition is the substance of things hoped for (results in all your hard work) and the evidence of things not seen (staying patient until you see results). Guaranteed. I want to encourage you, if you're exercising regularly, it IS working.

Continue to step out in faith and be patient. Do NOT grow weary with your exercise. Keep up the good work and stay in motion. Those results that you're after will surely come to pass. GUARANTEED. I don't know about you, but this news makes me want to EXERCISE.

Coconut Oil Craze
Day 168

rest
day

It's always fun watching food trends emerge. Coconut oil got my attention. It's one of the few foods that can be classified as a "super food." It has a unique combination of fatty acids that can profoundly affect your health. This includes weight loss, better brain function, and beauty/health benefits.

Coconut oil helps with fat loss. It has gotten a bad rap in the past because it contains saturated fat. It's one of the richest sources of saturated fats, BUT the difference is that fatty acids in our diet are long-chain fatty acids. Coconut oil has medium-chain fatty acids. These medium-chain acids metabolize differently. They go straight to the liver from the digestive tract, where they're used as a quick source of energy. It can increase your 24-hour energy expenditure by 5%. Who knew that coconut oil could be a healthy vehicle to help you burn more fat?

Regarding better brain function, ketones, which are byproducts of the breakdown of fats, play an important role in brain health. Boosting ketones can improve cognitive function.

Coconut oil also helps with your skin and hair. It acts as a wonderful moisturizer. It has good amounts of the antioxidant vitamin E, which is very protective. The positive antioxidant action provided by coconut oil helps stop damage to the tissues in our body. That can help with the aging process.

Keep in mind, fat is fat, and coconut oil is still high in calories, which can quickly add up around your waist. However, consider using coconut oil rather than your "go to" oil, just don't apply it too liberally.

When taking any new supplements, it's best to consult your doctor first. I encourage you to do your own research. This supplement could give your body the boost you need.

Is Caffeine Good or Bad?
Day 169

Before we discuss if caffeine is good or bad for you, I believe it's a personal matter. If you personally like caffeine's effects on your body, then it can be a good thing. If you personally dislike the effects caffeine has on your body, then it's probably not the wisest thing to drink.

Here are some advantages and disadvantages of caffeine.

Advantages:

Caffeine consumption can increase physical performance. Yes, it's true, there is evidence that caffeine can improve physical performance.

Caffeine consumption helps the body burn fat instead of carbohydrates. We are all going to burn more fat instead of carbohydrates if we continually exercise longer than 16 minutes. Caffeine can blunt the perception of "exercise pain," which can also boost endurance. This is why caffeine is found in almost every commercial fat-burning supplement.

Caffeine consumption is also good for heart health. Coffee can also reduce inflammation, and this helps prevent certain heart-related illnesses.

Disadvantages:

Caffeine can cause stomach problems. Some individuals are simply more sensitive than others. Drinking caffeinated drinks can irritate the lining of the small intestine, potentially leading to abdominal spasms, cramps, and elimination problems.

Caffeine can affect your sleep. Caffeine taken during the day may prevent you from falling asleep at night or it may shorten the normal length of your needed time of sleep.

Coffee can act as an unwanted diuretic. Drinking coffee can stimulate peristalsis, the process in the digestive tract that makes us head for the bathroom.

I encourage you to ask yourself, "Is caffeine really good for me? Am I sensitive, or is my body able to handle the caffeine in coffee, tea, or other caffeinated drinks?" Listen to your body, it speaks loudly if you let it.

Commit to an Adventure
Day 170

One of life's greatest guarantees, as you know it now, is headed for change. From hair color to strong opinions, all things will change, guaranteed. A determination to adapt to certain changes should include a commitment to keeping your heart healthy.

Without this determination to adapt, there is a lot to lose. The heart is the most important muscle in your body. If you don't have good heart health, it makes it extremely hard to do the simplest of tasks, especially as you age.

Remaining heart healthy requires a commitment, but I want to encourage you to make that commitment an adventure. Have fun with your fitness program. It's okay to take care of yourself. Your commitment to fitness, such as maintaining a healthy heart and body, will make everything else you want to do possible and in great physical condition.

God has the very hairs of our head numbered. He cares about your exercise program. Psalms 139:14 (NIV), "I praise you because I am fearfully and wonderfully made; your works are wonderful, I know that full well."

I challenge you to stay committed and be adventurous with your gift of health. Your heart will thank you and your quality of life will be proof.

Exercise and Chess ... A Similar Game
Day 171

I'm not a chess player, but what little I do know about the game is that there are similarities to successful fitness. The games of chess and exercise both involve strategic moves, they both take time to play, and they are both played to win.

To experience victory in your health and wellness, you must be strategic along the way. It's going to take some time, and you must know it's a battle up front. It's human nature to want to win at anything in life! Have you ever sat down to play a board game with young children? One of the first lessons in life is to teach a child to be a good sport (be happy for the winner, even if it's not you), play by the rules, and don't cheat!

The same is true with your health and wellness. When it comes to exercise, you've got to be a good sport because you WILL experience some setbacks, like the feeling that your hard work isn't paying off anymore. Life happens. It takes staying involved and being an active participant to WIN. Anything of great worth takes patience and time.

To succeed, you must play by the rules. The guidelines to fitness and nutrition must be followed in order to get the results we are all after. There are no shortcuts. Lastly, there must be strategy. Our bodies adapt very quickly to anything new, even to your exercise program and good nutrition. You must change things as you move forward.

Whether you are playing the game of chess or exercising, you're in it to win it. You might as well stay in the game, invest the time it takes, play by the rules, and win. Believe the best. There is a winner inside of us all.

Which Diet Works Best For Me?
Day 172

One of my new clients asked me to help her clean up her diet. For years, that's been an easy question for me. My recommendation has always been the nutrition of a bodybuilder. That's what I've known, and it works. But as I age in this industry, what worked five years ago doesn't necessarily work now.

I'd like to share a few different diets. We've got Paleo, Vegan, Weight Watchers, and Bodybuilder nutrition. Very vaguely they consist of:

Paleo Diet:
- Meat: Beef, lamb, chicken, turkey, pork, and others
- Fish and seafood: Salmon, trout, haddock, shrimp, shellfish, etc.
- Eggs: Choose free-range, pastured, or omega-3 enriched eggs
- Vegetables: Broccoli, kale, peppers, onions, carrots, tomatoes, etc.

Vegan Diet:
- Nuts, Nut Butters and Seeds
- Legumes
- Hemp, Flax, and Chia Seeds
- Tofu and Other Minimally Processed Meat Substitutes
- Calcium-Fortified Plant Milks and Yogurts
- Seaweed
- Nutritional Yeast
- Sprouted and Fermented Plant Foods

Food you eat on Weight Watchers:
- Fruits and Veggies
- Eggs, Skinless Chicken Breast, Fish, Seafood
- Corn, Beans, Peas

Food you eat on a Body builder Diet:
- Meats, poultry and fish: Sirloin steak, ground beef, pork tenderloin, venison, chicken breast, salmon, tilapia and cod
- Dairy: Yogurt, cottage cheese, low-fat milk, and cheese
- Grains: Bread, cereal, crackers, oatmeal, quinoa, popcorn and rice

My goal in sharing these different ways of eating is to open you up to the big world of nutrition and broaden your horizons. Why? Because maybe you've hit a plateau. Maybe you're stuck. Maybe you're experiencing that what you're eating isn't making you feel very good anymore. Or maybe you've never eaten right and want to try to better your nutrition.

Success is ALWAYS conquered outside your comfort zone.

185

What is Your Health and Wellness Perception?
Day 173

Do you look at the glass as half empty or half full? If your answer is half empty, I might conclude that you're looking at things in a negative way. If your answer is half full, my conclusion is you're looking at things in a positive way. A person's perception is their reality. That's why it's so important to have a right perception about your own health and wellness.

Most people's perception about their health and wellness is a "half empty" kind of perception. I'd like to encourage an accurate perception toward your individual fitness. I've seen people make AMAZING personal strides and still not acknowledge their accomplishments. When your body responds, it usually transpires in a way we're not expecting.

You may be at a place where you don't feel like anything good is happening physically. Be encouraged that you're literally adding years onto your life. Exercise helps the heart. Also, you're improving lung capacity and reducing the risk of heart disease and premature death.

A healthy heart will change any perception. I challenge you to embrace different fitness focal points as you continue on your journey. You can't get stuck on just weight loss. You must guard your perception.

Let's remember that many of the benefits from exercise are subtle. They may not be visible in the mirror. Your perception is key. Don't think for another second that exercise isn't working. If you're exercising, good things are happening. Have no doubt.

Your heart is strengthening. Your cholesterol levels and blood pressure are improving. Don't forget about how much easier you can perform daily tasks. Don't forget your increased energy levels are every bit as motivating, too. Let's squash the wrong perception once and for all. Buckle your seat belt for the long haul and enjoy your personal journey.

Laughter Burns Calories
Day 174

About twenty-five years ago, my mom, sister, and I were traveling from Tennessee to South Florida, and needless to say we were in the car for a while. I had recently read an article on how laughing burns a significant amount of calories.

To break a little boredom, I began to forcibly laugh. I kept laughing and laughing! At first I was only getting on my mom's and sister's nerves, but slowly and surely they began to laugh with me, and eventually we were all laughing so hard we cried.

We'd take a small break, and against their protests, I'd start the cycle all over again. Sure enough, they would join me and all of us filled the car with laughter. This went on for way too long, according to my sister and mom, BUT I wonder how many calories we burned.

Laughter is important. It's even written in the Bible. Proverbs 17:22 starts, "A happy heart is good medicine and a cheerful mind works healing…" Who knew laughter could be so powerful?

Sure, we need a balance of fun and responsibility, but too often we omit the fun part. If we're not emotionally balanced, our entire lives will be affected. Laughter can be instrumental in bringing healing to the body. Laughter is like internal jogging; it literally exercises our inner soul, bringing health to it.

You have homework from your trainer today. Find some kind of enjoyment in your life today while you work and perform the things you are supposed to do. Life is serious enough; let's not take ourselves too seriously, especially when we're alone. Laughter does the body good. It burns calories while being good medicine and is healthy, too.

Progress MUST Be Celebrated
Day 175

rest day

Have you ever been hard on yourself? Have you ever had thoughts like, "I don't like my stomach," "My legs are too fat," or "My arms look horrible" or similar self-defeating thoughts? Sometimes these thoughts can be consuming and tormenting. I've spent a lifetime beating myself up. I'm realizing I'm not alone.

The first thing we must do is find some progress. If you're doing one good thing toward better health, don't tell me you're not making any progress. If you're exercising a little, there is progress being made. If you're exercising a lot, there is progress being made. If you're making small steps to better eating, there is progress being made. If you're making major adjustments in your diet, there is progress being made.

Give it some thought; start seeking out your own personal progress. Thinking this way may feel very foreign. Becoming progress-focused must be intentional. If we don't become aware of the positive things that are taking place through making better choices, we'll become weakened in defeat.

Personal progress must be celebrated. You need to celebrate. Whether your celebration comes in the form of shopping for a new outfit or eating that one small sweet treat, the very act of celebration strengthens you. Set realistic goals that will keep you on track for rewarding yourself for a job well done.

Progress comes through making changes for the better. Making changes sometimes means you must face the truth of what you're doing wrong then being willing to learn better ways to do it. When you see the truth about yourself, you become aware of the things you need to work on. That's growth.

Be kind to yourself in the process of growth. I challenge you to look for your progress and celebrate.

Me, Me, Me, Me, Me
Day 176

Let's face it, we're on our own minds a lot. So how do you see yourself? What thoughts about yourself have your attention today? Are you thinking, "Wow, I'm pretty fit, but I wish I was taller," or "I'm smart but I wish I was thinner," or "If only…"

If we're not careful, one wrong self-image thought can wreck our whole day. What a waste of precious unrecoverable time and energy. So here's a challenge — instead of looking at yourself with such a critical eye, why not look at yourself with a thankful eye?

Look at all you're doing. Look at all you have. Look at all you're capable of. For the most part, you're probably quite healthy, and without a doubt I feel certain you're probably very smart.

So when your feet hit the floor tomorrow morning, first thing I want you to do is count your fingers and toes. If they're all there, then celebrate with a smile in your heart because you're off to a good start.

Got food to eat for breakfast? Celebrate! Got a job? Celebrate! Going to work out with me today or this week? Double celebrate!

You are healthy. You are an exerciser or may even be in an elite group known as fitness enthusiasts. Remember to be thankful. Remember to celebrate. You might as well celebrate things to be thankful for since you've got yourself on your mind.

Let's always remember to look at the glass half full.

Just Be
Day 177

I have been watching the news quite often lately, which is out of my normal routine. Some people might think I'm putting my head in the sand by not being a big news watcher, but the truth is, I find the news hard to handle mentally. When I overload my mind with current events, I feel hopeless, and I begin to fear things that are truly out of my control.

Having all this news in my head, I've started thinking about how to "Just Be" in this world today. If we take on the world's stress, it will affect our individual well-being. Furthermore, our perception becomes our reality, and so if we have a hopeless perception of today's tumultuous world, we'll find it hard to "Just Be."

One way we can "Just Be" is to stay physically fit. Good health allows us to better handle life's stress and demands. Therefore, the best gift we can give ourselves is the gift of fitness. Fitness keeps us mentally sharp and ready to handle whatever the future holds.

A second way to "Just Be" is to pray. We CAN pray for things that are too big to handle and have faith we are furthering the good of the world. By bowing my head to pray about world affairs, I can have a supernatural peace afterwards.

Do you have your health and wellness in order so you can "Just Be" in this world? The Bible tells us in 1 Thessalonians 5:6, "You must be on your guard, not asleep like others." So, we must stay alert and clear-headed. We do this by staying fit, strong, and prepared for the battle at hand. We cannot lose heart at such a time is this. It's time that we "Just Be."

Fantastic Fitness Featuring Client's Testimony
Day 178

Success, success, and more success. As we know, health and wellness success is hard to come by. Today, I'd like to share the biggest motivator: a true, real, live, personal testimony.

Here is my client's story:

"In my younger days, I was extremely active. Like most people, I worked out less and sat down more as I aged. Having a sedentary occupation didn't help my waistline. Neither did my diet.

I decided I should change direction and had a physical for the first time in years. My doctor gave me some obvious news. I was overweight. In order to prevent health issues, I should alter my lifestyle. I dramatically cut my carbohydrate intake by following the Paleo diet. I felt so good that I chose Paleo for another 30 days. In addition, I starting going to the gym after receiving encouragement from a friend/co-worker of mine.

I began a regular gym schedule of Monday, Thursday, Saturday, and Sunday. Having a regular gym partner is a tremendous motivation. I wanted to track my results, so I weighed and measured myself every week.

One month later, I've lost a total of 20 pounds and 15 inches spread between my neck, chest, waist, and hips. In addition to the weight and inches lost, I am no longer winded when I go out for a walk, I feel stronger, and in general I have more energy.

I know it took years to put the weight and inches on so I don't expect it to come off overnight. While these results are encouraging, I've set long-term goals for myself and I'm not content with where I'm at yet. This is just the beginning of a long journey!"

I challenge you to continually seek true contentment with yourself and your fitness.

Every Little Bit Matters
Day 179

Do you always give your 100%? All or nothing is the way I roll, too. This motto isn't true, however, when it comes to exercise. Instead, we must grasp the mindset of every little bit we do matters.

I'd like to address those of you who are about to give up on reaching your fitness goals. As you do life, things change—mentally and physically. Think about that. Do you think or look like you did twenty years ago? We have to manage our expectations.

Every little bit matters when your goal is to keep fitness a big part of your life for a long period of time. Don't drop out of fitness because you got distracted by "more important things" in life. Don't stop because you feel impatient with trying to meet your fitness goals and don't believe it's even worth trying anymore.

Below are some small things you can try to keep fitness in your life.

Go hiking with a friend every week. Hiking gets you out of your typical routine and gets you moving.

Go dancing. I had quality porch time with my 76 year-old daddy when he wanted to learn country line-dancing. Dancing is a wonderful way to stay fit and keep moving.

Go outdoors to do your favorite activities. Walk your dog, take your children to the park (and play with them), ride horseback, or go kayaking. Being active on the water is healing to the soul.

Do anything. Take the stairs, do extra chores around the house, or walk to the mailbox. Remember, every little bit matters.

I've heard it said the secret to getting ahead is getting started. I encourage you to get started and stay engaged.

THIRD QUARTER
Daily Inspirations for Fitness

It Gets Tough in the Interim
Days 180 - 270

**Scan the QR Code for each day
to take you to a companion
YouTube Video Workout**

Are You Ready to Rumble?
Day 180

It's 11:30 p.m. on a Friday night; you're alone and bored. What do you do – Head to the fridge, or head to the closet to see what clothes fit for the first time in a long time? That's the challenge one of my clients faced recently.

She made a great decision. She really wanted to eat her boredom away. She had made lots of headway in the gym training for months, so she really didn't want to sabotage all of her hard work. She found herself heading straight to the closet to try on those desired clothes that hadn't fit for a long time. Much to her amazement, they fit! She was so excited that she called and woke up her mother to share her great news.

It's a battle out there against everything that's combating for your attention. The question is: Are you ready to rumble? Are you ready to duke it out and overcome the plethora of temptations and excuses? Be prepared.

Preparation is key to combating temptations: lay your workout clothes out the night before so you don't have to fumble around in the morning looking for them. If you're bored and feel yourself reaching for a Twinkie, be alert: grab a book or a glass of water, or go for a short, brisk walk.

I challenge you to have an activity in mind that is the opposite of your weakness. Don't give in to the obstacles that are sure to come. Making these small choices for better health can keep you away from a life of inactivity and destructive eating habits.

Be prepared, awake, and alert at all times and you will experience a life of victory by making one good choice at a time. Be ready to rumble.

Standing -vs- Sitting
Day 181

rest
day
It seems not long ago, driving home from church, my 17-year-old said, "Momma, I didn't eat the chips and drink the soda tonight in small group, because I remembered you saying every single good choice toward better health matters."

Boy oh boy, I felt immediate conviction. I had food on my mind, thinking about what I was going to devour in the fridge, and it wasn't salad. Even worse, it wasn't because I was hungry, but because I was bored.

I'm excited to share I wrote in victory that next morning. I talked myself into making a small good choice (with the help of my daughter) to not eat out of boredom. You may be asking, "Why this silly little story?" It led me to share that the small choice to STAND more than SIT reaps great rewards.

Again, "Making the effort to STAND more than SIT reaps great rewards." The caloric difference of standing has a much higher heart rate, which adds up to burning about 50 calories more per hour than sitting.

Standing will help you lose 8 to 20 pounds over the course of a year through making standing adjustments for 4 hours each day. Not only does it generate more calories to stand, but making standing adjustments versus sitting has more benefits.

*Standing improves posture while excessive sitting can exacerbate postural problems and inflexibility.

*Standing reduces aches and pains while excessive sitting may compress the spine and may tighten the chest, shoulder, and neck muscles.

*Standing more often contributes to an overall better sense of well-being and health while sitting can cause you to become lethargic.

Remember, every SMALL choice you make matters, whether making a point to not eat when you're bored or to STAND for a while. Victory comes in small choices.

196

Body Composition Options
Day 182

rest day

What's body composition? It's the proportion of fat, muscle, and bone of an individual's body, expressed as a percentage of body fat and percentage of lean body mass. Conversely, scale weight is just one measurement of a total mass and doesn't compute muscle, fat, bones, or fluids.

I attended a continuing education workshop this past weekend, and we discussed the types of body composition options:

• The Bod Pod: The Bod Pod looks like a giant egg. You sit in the egg while the technician uses a computer-operated scanner to scan your body as you sit in the giant egg. The Bod Pod is fairly new, having been formally introduced in 1994. It took first place in underwater weighing for being the "Most Accurate" way of measuring your body composition.

• Hydrostatic Underwater Weighing: This method is done by weighing on land first. Next, the person will get into a large tank of water, and while sitting on a special scale, is lowered underwater and asked to expel all air from the lungs and remain motionless while the underwater weight is measured.

• Lange Calipers: Back in my day, the Lange Calipers were the thing. I was happy to learn that they still are a very good resource for body fat measurements. Lange Calipers are used to measure four body sites and then calculate those particular sites to find your body fat measurements.

• Other methods, such as infrared, body composition scales, and other body composition devices, can also be surprisingly accurate. My instructor this past weekend (a professional swimmer), did the Hydrostatic underwater weighing. That same day she stepped on a body composition scale, and to her surprise, it was as accurate as her underwater results.

Don't get fixed on a fictitious, unattainable, number on a scale..... Seek out body composition options.

Age-Related Muscle Loss
Day 183

Age-related muscle loss is a real thing, and it can start at a relatively young age. By the time you enter your third decade of life, your age-related muscle is on the decline. From then on, you can lose an average of seven pounds of muscle each decade unless you take steps to prevent it.

Evidence does suggest the aging of your cells can indeed be slowed, and in some cases, even reversed, with the appropriate diet and exercise. It's important to realize your daily activities play a key role in this process. What you eat, when you eat, and how you exercise all translate into genetic activities that dictate the speed at which your body ages.

While we know muscle loss is a natural effect associated with aging, it doesn't have to be an inevitable fate. A healthy and active 60-year-old can have the muscle mass of a 30-year-old. On the other hand, a sedentary middle-aged person may have the muscle quality of a 70-year-old.

In our forties, our metabolism slows down and the loss of muscle mass inevitably becomes a natural part of aging during this time. Those striving for optimal health and wellness during this decade should fit cardio training into their routine every week. Resistance training is also a must because it has been proven that cardio workouts burn more calories than strength training, but remember, you need both.

If this truth has motivated you to work out, make sure you first consult your doctor (especially if you're older). Your doctor can determine how much exercise and what specific exercise plan is best for you. Aging is NOT for the weak at heart.

FACTS into ACTion
Day 184

One thing is true - you can't ignore facts about the human body.

If you're looking for magic, there's no magic to good health. As technology advances and lots of new methods come on the market, some things can be found to be a great aid in helping you look your best. But nothing is magic.

You body is fearfully and wonderfully made. The functional design of your body is supernatural. You body is smart. It catches on quickly to the demands you place on it. One fact that must be placed into action is the body needs movement and to be challenged for positive growth.

If you've faced physical trauma, like an unfortunate car accident, surgery, broken bones, etc., a big part of recovery is movement. During the recovery process, there's always some kind of challenging part for specific healing and growth.

Another fact that needs action: you must burn more calories than you consume to lose weight. This truth will never change. Also, if you don't burn your food due to a sedentary lifestyle, you're put at risk for many health problems and decreased mobility.

During exercise sessions, you're literally turning your body into an efficient machine that becomes a calorie burner - increasing your metabolism and making your body able to rid itself of excess calories. Through exercise, your body becomes well regulated, not wanting to hang on to extra calories.

On top of these great facts, exercising enhances brain clarity; that keeps you sharp for your job plus alert for important appointments. This information should spur you into action and staying motivated to pursue better health.

Always focus on being vigorous in making the choice to exercise. Stay encouraged to carry on and stay fit. I challenge you to take ACTION and act upon every opportunity for movement.

The Most Important Muscle
Day 185

I just returned from a weekend of continuing education, and I was reminded of the importance that exercise has on your heart. Our goals, as unique as we all are, are understandably vastly different. But there is one vital factor that we all have in common, and that is our hearts.

Did you know that your heart is a muscle? Yep, it's a muscle. Some people might think it's an organ, but it's not; it's a muscle. Over this past weekend in class, a woman raised her hand and asked the question, "Why do we need to know this as fitness professionals? No one really cares about how the heart works; they just want to work out." Sure, that's probably true. You don't go to exercise class to get a lecture on your heart. You go to exercise class to get a workout. But, I'll bet the next time you do train, you might be motivated differently to push yourself, knowing that your heart is getting a workout, too.

When you work out, your heart (like all other muscles in the body) becomes stronger and in turn affects your blood pressure. During classes, I love to see my amazing clients begin to breathe hard. This "labored breathing" is like good medicine. I know they are challenging themselves enough to reap the benefits of not only the toned bodies we all desire, but a healthy, happy heart, too.

Our hearts aren't usually on a person's mind heading out the door to exercise class. We take the heart for granted very easily. If the heart doesn't work properly, we have major health problems. If it stops ticking, we stop ticking. Embrace your weekly routine, knowing you are taking care of the most important muscle in your body.

Keep up the Good Work
Day 186

'Keep up the good work' sounds so cliché, but it's so true! As you keep up the good work of exercise, you'll soon find a theme developing in your life called consistency. The only thing that brings lasting results in this fitness journey is consistency.

This is a cause-and-effect world we live in, so you can't expect any improvements if you don't put in the time and effort to get them. If you're exercising regularly, you are doing good work. If you're not, I'm here to tell you it's never too late to begin. We all want to feel better, have more energy, and live longer.

The health benefits of regular exercise and physical activity are hard to ignore, regardless of your age, sex, or physical ability. Exercise can aid in all of these common desires we share. Consistent exercise aids in weight loss. It lowers your risk for health problems and improves moods. Regular exercisers burn more fat when they work out on a regular basis. Consistency develops higher levels of fitness and opens the door to more exercise options, avoiding boredom and burnout. Muscle content has more anti-aging impact than stress or genetics.

The biggest reason to keep up the good work is activities of daily life improve. Americans' sedentary lifestyles have made daily tasks challenging. More and more people are turning to their doctors for a pill to give them more energy.

No matter where you are in your health and wellness journey, stay consistent. Through all the highs, lows, and changes that a health and wellness journey brings, keeping up the good work is the only place you can find lasting results. I challenge you to take hold and make your exercise program work for you. Keep up the good work.

Increasing Your Resistance is Necessary
Day 187

As a new exerciser begins resistance training, their strength soon grows. Initially challenged by five-pound dumbbells, before long those same weights look like "baby rattles." The committed exerciser soon finds themselves stronger and stronger, ready to seek out a greater challenge.

The strength gains of my clients is very rewarding to me. This increase in strength is usually the first sign of progress. In the beginning, these gains happen quickly. It's good to stay aware of the gains so you know to increase weight.

Here are some signs that indicate it's time to increase your weight:

When your current weight isn't a challenge. Strength training is meant to be challenging. The whole point is to "overload" your muscles so they get stronger.

When you could go forever. Each strength-training exercise you do should cause you to feel muscle "fatigue" within 15 repetitions. Muscle fatigue feels like you couldn't possibly do another repetition in good form. If you can do more than 15 reps in good form, it's time for more weight.

When you've never increased your weight. When you first started strength training, the weight you lifted was a starting weight. Continuing to increase weight is essential to getting the most out of your workouts.

The goal in strength training is to fatigue the muscles. Completing the exact number of reps is secondary, but all too often, people become too focused on reaching a certain number of reps without paying attention to adding more weight for fatigue.

You'll have good days and bad days. Sometimes you'll feel like the Incredible Hulk, where the weight feels as light as a feather. Other days you'll feel like Pee Wee Herman, when what was easy two days ago feels like a ton today. I challenge you to adjust accordingly.

The Tough Keep Going
Day 188

rest day

Some days a pep talk is necessary. When you've been exercising and eating right for years, accomplishing a lot of goals you've set for yourself, it can feel quite monotonous at times, feeling like you don't want to do this health and wellness thing anymore.

The only way to stay successful in this health and wellness journey is to keep going. I had a client share how she lost to her desired weight through a weight-loss program. She was ready to quit. She achieved her desired weight and thought that was her arrival point.

There's no arrival point in fitness. We must accept that health and wellness is a constant journey. The key is to KEEP going. When life gets tough or when you hit a milestone in fitness, it's more incentive to keep going.

A fitness journal helps you stick to your healthy goals. Journaling will help you handle your victories and defeats in stride. It will keep your mind focused on daily tasks to continually set you up for success. It may also expose any bad habits you might be falling into. For example, maybe you're gaining weight because you're eating the same but stopped exercising.

Try starting your exercise week on Monday. This sets the psychological pattern for the week. Monday workouts are the hardest workouts, but the sense of accomplishment sets the stage for more workouts.

It's good not to skip exercise two days in a row. On the day you skipped, it's good to start thinking about your next workout. Keep your fitness on your mind. No matter how inconvenient your exercise time can be, you shouldn't allow too many days to go by without putting those exercise shoes on to hit it again.

We are the tough. By golly we WILL keep going.

Extreme Caution
Day 189

Being extreme, regardless of the topic or situation, is being at one end of the spectrum, which is not close to being moderate. In some areas, to be extreme may be considered okay. However, in a fitness journey, extremes are to be avoided; moderation is our goal.

My heart breaks when I see an adult or child who is eating unhealthy food to an extreme, keeping them from their best life. I can relate because I ate to an extreme that kept me from doing the things that I wanted to do, too. My exercise addiction kept obesity at bay. It's made me very sensitive to people who've taken on an extreme lifestyle, opposite of enjoying a life of health and wellness.

The same goes when I see a person in the gym that is literally skin and bones, madly running from one piece of equipment to another at breakneck speed trying to burn that one more percent of body fat they don't even have to burn. Both extremes are heartbreaking and life threatening. Since moderation is our goal, let's be reminded of some basic guidelines of exercise for healthy adults under the age of 65:

- Do moderately intense cardio 30 minutes a day, 5 days a week.
- Do 8 to 10 strength training exercises with 8 to 12 reps of each twice a week.

We all have a tendency to be extreme about one thing or another. Be cautious of any extremes that might be present in your life that are trying to drag you from one end of the rope to the other. I challenge you to be aware at all times and strive to remain moderate. Your body will thank you!

Does Calorie Restriction Really Work?
Day 190

Yes, in order to lose weight, restricting calories must be applied. You have to eat less and burn more calories to lose weight. This truth to losing weight sometimes seems hopeless when finding the perfect method. I'd like to encourage you to keep weight loss simple, not fanatical.

Here are some fad methods to be cautious of:

The low-carb diet. A low-carb plan has allowed many of us to feel the thrill of slipping back into our skinny jeans. But the low-carb diet worked for one simple reason: we ate less.

Setting your daily calorie limit too low. Your body thinks you're starving, and you lose too much too fast. Instead of burning calories, it conserves them in the form of fat. As many as half of the pounds you drop during crash dieting comes from muscle rather than fat.

All fad diets that promise they are the best. The problem with these methods are when you go back to any normality of eating food, you gain all your weight back. Fad diets aren't sustainable.

Simple ways to create a calorie deficit:

Do something every day. Making a daily decision to eat one less thing or move your body for ten minutes sets your metabolism up for fueling your muscles properly, which gives you lasting weight loss.

Standardize your eating habits in eating the same way every day. This will keep your calories in check. Make sure your food choices consist of fiber and protein. These burn off slowly, which helps you avoid hunger pangs.

Eat slowly and give your body enough time to digest so you can properly decide when you're full.

I challenge you to make simple choices and stay away from the stress of restricting your calories in a dramatic way that won't last.

Activity in my Home State
Day 191

I did some research about eight years ago on activity and inactivity in the United States, and my home state of Tennessee didn't rank too well. Recently, I was curious to see if our lovely, beautiful state has gotten any better in our fitness ranking. To my disappointment, we were even worse than before! We were the 49th most inactive state in America.

I then wondered what criteria makes a state inactive and unfit. I found that sitting is a big problem. Minimal to no movement is a detriment to an individual's overall health. There are too many inactive adults, and they may not know how much it affects their health. Studies have proven that being physically active helps you sleep better, feel better, and reduce your risk for obesity, heart disease, type 2 diabetes, and some cancers.

We Tennesseans must remain hopeful and begin to change our inactive community by encouraging active lifestyles. Health and wellness is a gift, not a chore. Let us go forward in movement and reverse our state's statistics. I remain hopeful for our awesome state of Tennessee to improve its fitness level. Let's do our part and influence the people in our circles to move and get active!

Do You Eat to Live or Live to Eat?
Day 192

This question is by far the biggest struggle I've faced my whole fitness career. I don't understand why something so simple is so hard. You feed your body food as fuel and you live a great, healthy life. Or you can struggle like me and think about food far too much. It seems I'm always wasting too much brain space on my next meal.

If you are a person who lives to eat, I'm sure you've experienced frustration with eating. The food and diet industry continues to offer consumers a variety of diet pills, meal plans, and weight-loss solutions.

Eating should be a pleasurable and enjoyable time of day, not a time when negative thoughts overtake the natural process of food for fuel. The first step toward natural, healthy eating and positive lifestyle change is to create awareness about your eating style.

Eating styles tend to fall into two major categories: mindful calorie eaters (eat to live), or intuitive eaters (live to eat). The number one goal for eating and changing habits is to first recognize obsessive thoughts related to eating. The aim is to bring awareness and intention to your eating habits, which include thoughts, actions, and behaviors.

Discovering what eating style fits your lifestyle, goals, and personality is essential for success. Which one are you? Do you have the eating style of a calorie eater or an intuitive eater? Begin by asking yourself the following three questions:

1. How do I currently eat?
2. Does it help or hinder my progress, thoughts, or habits?
3. What habits can I adopt to create a healthier change?

The ultimate goal is to awaken awareness. I encourage you to learn your eating style and preference. This will help get you set up for success in achieving future goals.

Exercise With a Purpose
Day 193

Have you got a "willy nilly" or "what difference does it make" attitude regarding your workout? Or do you go to the gym with a purpose in mind, knowing every time you're there it makes a difference? It's true, everything you do makes a difference.

All of us have fitness goals in mind. To achieve them we must exercise with a purpose. An aimless attempt will only leave you feeling frustrated and discouraged. If you find yourself wandering from one thing to another and not being really focused, stop for a moment and gather your thoughts. Encouraging yourself and knowing what you're doing daily is making a difference. It IS making you better.

Your efforts don't have you idling; you're getting somewhere. So when you think it doesn't matter, know that it does. When you're in limbo, try asking yourself, "Do I or don't I workout today?" Always pick "do" because "don't" never accomplishes anything. Every day and every effort matters.

Fitness has its individual degrees and levels of struggle. Don't diminish, belittle, or judge yourself in your struggle. Just because your struggle is different than your "fit friend," don't perceive them as better than you just because they don't appear to be struggling like you. Exercise is personal. I challenge you to exercise with a purpose, knowing it IS making a difference.

Why in the World Am I Not Losing Weight?
Day 194

Have you ever set out to lose weight? It may have been for a special occasion, or perhaps you were tired of carrying around extra weight. These attempts to lose weight typically come to a crashing end. Most people's quests to lose weight end in frustration because little or no progress has been made. Truth be known, better health and wellness can't be accomplished through preparing for one special occasion or jumping in with high expectations.

Sure, you might find some success, but true long-term success is found through a continual pursuit of exercise, consistency, and moderation.

Consistency is hard to maintain in such an "I want it now" society. When your body doesn't respond quickly enough, being consistent falls by the wayside. Striving for better health takes dedication and hard work. When you're struggling to lose weight, your body goes through a resistant period of not budging. Consistency in your efforts is key to breaking through the resistance.

Moderation is a needed boundary. Most of us eat like we drive our cars; both are pretty thoughtless, automatic acts. When driving, not much thought goes into stopping at a red light. The same thing applies when we eat; not much thought goes into what we put into our mouths. Simply giving some thought to what you're eating is a great way to help you not go overboard and set yourself back. Also, practicing portion control is a great way to stay in control.

If you're trying to lose weight and it isn't going according to plan, do a self-check. Sometimes we have to encourage ourselves to continue on with our exercise plan, consistency, and moderation. I challenge you to believe you can lose weight because you're not going to quit.

Put Your War Clothes On
Day 195

I often think about how we ALL want that perfect, hot body. We ALL realize the hard work and dedication it takes. We must realize we're in battle.

This brings me to a story when I first got into the personal training business. In the mid '80's, when only the wealthy could afford a trainer, I arrived at one of my client's homes. Walking up to the front door, I was greeted by their assistant. I walked in as my client was descending in a gorgeous glass elevator. When the elevator opened, she came out and greeted me with bare feet. She had just received a pedicure.

This privileged client of mine had the wealth to afford any amenity, including me. What she didn't realize was the amenity I offered came with an element she wasn't dressed or ready for...the battle. She had no idea; she had to put her WAR clothes on.

Exercise is a war zone. Be ready. You've got to be ready for the battle (workout). You've got to be prepared both physically and mentally. You must be ready to sweat, cry tears of joy, and be in it for the hard work it takes to achieve goals.

I'm going to dress you for battle.

WIN: Whatever you set out to do for exercise, decide before the excuses come. You'll win every time.

ACHIEVE: Before each workout, decide that you are your own competition. Set small goals to attain during each workout. Compete with your personal record.

RETURN: This rodeo never ends. You must decide to return to exercise over and over again.

Do you have your war clothes on? Health and wellness are a battlefield. There's no time for a pedicure before you train; you've got to show up prepared. Be ready for war.

Summer Wear
Day 196

How do the words "bathing suits, shorts, skirts, short-sleeved shirts, picnics, boating, beaches, or pool parties" make you feel? Some people don't even partake in any of the above due to fear of how they look. Body insecurity is a real issue. You may be battling body insecurity due to being overweight or having a distorted self-image. Whatever the case, this is a real issue.

Exercise can help body insecurities. Very rarely do you look in the mirror and say, "Wow, I look great!" The good news is exercise does create a sense of accomplishment that brings confidence. You mustn't be so focused on the way you look or you'll never venture out of your home. You need to resist being controlled by your negative self thoughts or by what you think others think of you. Your goal must be to cultivate a healthy self-image that sets you free to do summer things that require summer wear.

Don't allow a low self-image to keep you inside the house. You're missing out by saying no to all that your summer entails. If you're exercising regularly and putting effort into eating healthy, then you have every right to walk with confidence. You can enjoy a pair of shorts. You can allow yourself to wear a short-sleeved shirt or swimsuit, confidently.

I challenge you to not get stuck inside the house because of body insecurities. Be determined to discover all the summer fun you've missed out on. We all have imperfect bodies. Everyone's health and wellness requires maintenance and takes constant work. You must remember — exercising has no arrival point. You might as well find peace and enjoy along your lifetime fitness journey.

Don't let life pass you by. Enjoy your summer wear. You've earned it.

Are Sports Drinks Necessary?
Day 197

Often when people begin an exercise program, they think sports drinks, such as Powerade® or Gatorade®, are good for them anytime. This myth couldn't be further from the truth. Sports drinks are for athletes that exercise for an extended duration such as triathlons, Iron Mans or marathons.

In some cases, if you've been really sick and need the extra calories and sodium, replenishing sports drinks serve a good purpose in your recovery. Drinks like these are NOT good for the regular exerciser, especially if you are just starting out in an exercise program. I think the misconception comes from advertisement.

If you've watched any kind of TV, I'm sure you've come across a Powerade® or Gatorade® commercial that inspires you to want to workout and afterwards drink a sports drink. Throughout the day, and in particular when we exercise, our bodies lose fluids, leaving us in a depleted state in need of water.

Water is the better replenisher for the average exerciser. This is true because of the sodium and carbohydrates that are in sports drinks. If we want to lose weight, we are trying to create a caloric deficiency, so the last thing we need is to drink more calories and hold extra sodium. Even if you're an avid exerciser, you still don't need the extra calories.

Water can serve as a great tool to get your body moving and rid itself of toxins. Water is so good for us. Let us encourage each other. Don't be fooled by those awesome sports drink commercials again. Remember, water will always be the ultimate replenisher.

Train Your Body Evenly
Day 198

I'm all about pumping some iron. I love the feeling, the benefits, and the results. Everybody has a favorite muscle group they like to train. Having a favorite is fine, but what we must not lose sight of is that your favorite muscles have opposing muscles. These opposing muscles need your attention, too!

Opposing muscles are the muscles that do the opposite of the muscle that is working. For example, when a person performs a bicep curl, the opposing muscle group is the triceps. Many people simply don't realize the importance of good muscle balance. If you're not sure of the body's muscles and their opposing groups, here are some very basic groups that need to be trained either together or within your weekly fitness regime.

Pectoral muscles (chest) oppose the *latissimus dorsi* (back). When pectoral muscles are tight from excessive focus and not spending enough time on the lats, range of motion at the shoulder can be affected.

Quadriceps (thighs) oppose the hamstrings (back of legs). An over-development of the quadriceps in conjunction with an underdevelopment of the hamstrings can compromise posture and one's gait due to the muscular imbalance.

Bicep muscles oppose the triceps muscle. It's common to see over-developed bicep muscles and underdeveloped triceps muscle. Having overdeveloped biceps can limit extension at the elbow if the triceps are underdeveloped, causing decreased range of motion and even pain in the elbow joints.

Abdominals (tummy) and erector spine muscles (lower back). The abdominal muscles are for core stabilization, but balancing work on the abs with work on muscles that create back extension is important for overall core strength and muscular balance around the spine. Staying in balance keeps injury or chronic pain away. Let's keep our bodies happy and in balance! :)

Change
Day 199

Have you ever been in a wonderful season of life you didn't want to change? Like when you were in the honeymoon stage of marriage, for instance, or starting a family, enjoying the success of your children, or just landing your dream job. Maybe it's the opposite. You're in a season of life you desperately wanted to change. Like a divorce, for example, or bad report from the doctor, the loss of a loved one, or having a rebellious child.

Even if your life is stress-free, your physical body will definitely change. I've learned through the years, most people become impatient with change. They fail to realize the time it takes for things (good or bad) to develop into change. Physical body tone, weight loss, weight gain, endurance, and increased strength will all change in time. How you eat, what you do for cardiovascular and resistance training will also change. Whatever season of life, things are bound to change.

Here are two effective lifestyles adapted for different seasons of life.

Example #1 - My personal plan (in my fifties):

- I eat moderately because it's best for my body.
- I do five days of cycling for 45 minutes. I started three-mile casual walks for active enjoyment.
- I do five days of modified resistance training for 30 minutes.

Example #2 - My daughter's plan (in her early twenties):

- She has an extremely strict diet of high protein, very low carbohydrates, and two protein shakes daily.
- She does extremely intense cardio six days a week.
- She lifts heavy weights intensely five to six days a week.

Comparing the two plans, you can see the differences due to age, interests, and limitations. When the changes of a new day come, I encourage you to make lemonade out of any lemons life may throw your way.

Exercise When?
Day 200

There is a particular time of day that's best for you to exercise depending on your individuality and your internal clock. For instance, if you're a morning person, 7:00 p.m. workouts wouldn't be your most effective choice. The opposite is true if you're a night person; 4:00 a.m. workouts wouldn't be your best time for challenging exercise. Unless you're working out at your best exercise time, it can feel like a chore and its purpose can be misunderstood. Exercise should be an enjoyed part of life.

Everyone has an internal clock. Your internal clock is a certain circadian rhythm governed by the twenty-four hour pattern of the Earth's rotation. This rhythm influences body functions such as heart rate, body temperature, and hormone levels. All of these bodily functions play a role in your body's readiness for exercise.

It's important to know your body's own circadian rhythm. We all have different rhythms. In fact, we're each born with a particular rhythm or chronotype which we have to figure out. So are you an owl exerciser or a lark exerciser? Owls are more alert during the evenings, while larks are more alert in the mornings.

If you're a beginner, sometimes this internal clock is hard to read. It's good to have a scheduled exercise time to motivate you as you learn your own body rhythms. Set a time and try it. If you find that you hate your scheduled time, your body might be telling you that you have a different internal rhythm than you originally thought.

Learning our chronotypes will enable us to decide the best time of day to exercise. There are many options from which to choose. So let's not get caught up in excuses and learn to exercise at our best time.

What Exactly Are Super Foods?
Day 201

If optimal health is your goal, your diet must be addressed. Your physical health is a direct reflection of what you put into your body and how you live your life. It's good to know there are certain foods that are easy to add to your diet that carry rich nutrients to improve your health.

These particular foods are called "super foods." There are four super foods that can offer a wide range of essential nutrients that can easily be integrated into a balanced diet.

Eggs are relatively inexpensive and are an amazing source of high-quality nutrients that many people are deficient in, especially high-quality protein and fat. A single egg contains nine essential amino acids, one of the highest quality proteins.

Kale is an inexpensive vegetable that provides an excellent source of multiple vitamins and other nutrients, including Vitamin A (which contains calcium), Vitamin B (which contains iron), and Vitamin C (which is part of its chlorophyll).

Raw almonds contain mostly polyunsaturated and monounsaturated fats, which are good fats that promote healthy cholesterol levels. They have zero trans fats, as long as they're processed properly.

Wild Alaskan salmon is among the most recommended foods by registered dietitians for its outstanding nutritional benefits, which include high levels of omega-3 (with DHA and EPA). Most people are desperately lacking omega-3 in their diets. Registered dietitians typically recommend eating salmon one or two times per week, as it is an excellent source of essential animal-based omega-3 fats (EPA and DHA), antioxidants, and high-quality protein.

You now have some easy suggestions for healthy, nutrient-rich foods to add to your diet. These small power-packed foods will help you stay feeling great. Don't grow weary in doing good. You shall surely reap a happy belly … happy body.

Anchor In
Day 202

I was up early this morning praying and thinking about life. I wondered about what people do in their daily lives to feel anchored. Have you ever thought about what anchors you? Does your faith or seeing your spouse's smiling face keep you grounded? Is it watching your children excel or knowing they are home safe and sound?

Pertaining to health and wellness, maybe your anchor is going to the gym every day before work, doing a daily home workout, or meeting a friend regularly for an afternoon walk. It can be a particular something you eat or the ounces of water you drink in a day.

Anchor is defined as a person or thing that provides stability or confidence in an otherwise uncertain situation. This stuck out to me because we all know that life is uncertain. Health and wellness can definitely be an anchor in the uncertainty of life.

Exercise provides stability. It is a very powerful "drug" that does naturally what many scientists in the pharmaceutical world have been creating for decades. Maintaining a sense of physical balance is invaluable in feeling grounded and supported. Physical balance allows you to move safely from one place to another or to stand in place without feeling like you're going to teeter over.

Exercise provides credence to control and improvement in your overall well-being. Your productivity will improve and your mind will clear when you exercise regularly. Very often, what you thought was a major problem before exercising will disappear afterwards.

Who knew stability was a benefit of a health and wellness journey? Exercise can be an anchor that keeps you in the right frame of mind and puts some vigor in your step. So get anchored in with exercise.

Lies, Lies, and More Lies
Day 203

rest day Have you ever thought about how life is lived in a realistic manner, but there's this unseen unrealistic expectation of living life idealistically? For instance, Facebook is a pretty good example of an idealistic life versus a realistic life. Another example is the court system; they handle people's realistic lives based on an idealistic viewpoint.

These realistic and idealistic points of view hold true in the fitness arena, too. We all have idealistic points of view of what getting in shape looks like. We have high hopes and movie star dreams about all that we want to accomplish when we set out to become fit. Then, we soon learn the realistic things that happen to our bodies aren't measuring up to the ideal image we had in mind.

When reality hits us, disappointment sets in. Disappointment leads us to believe lies, lies, and more lies. If disappointment isn't dealt with, quitting is next.

Today, I'd like to talk about idealistic versus realistic fitness goals.

• An idealistic goal is to get washboard abs. A realistic goal is to lose inches.

• An idealistic goal is to get rid of cellulite. Realistically, cellulite can be reduced, but there's no way to completely eliminate cellulite.

• An idealistic goal is to get hyper-focused on losing a specific amount of weight. Realistically, your body has a certain ratio of fat, muscle, bone mass, and such; don't get stuck on a scale number.

• An idealistic goal is we often have a model-like image of what we want to look like. Realistically, we can never change the genetics of our bodies to be what they can't physically be.

You don't have time to focus on what will never be. Don't believe the lies, but instead be determined to work toward being all you can be.

Pep Talk Cheer
Day 204

Sometimes you can't count on others to cheer you on. You have to be able to cheer yourself on. Even in a room full of people, it's still possible to feel alone and in need of a pep talk. We must be able to build up and encourage ourselves in the things we are capable of doing.

Let's take some time today to cheer ourselves on. To do so, we need the reminder that it's not being arrogant or prideful, but it is the very thing needed and necessary when we feel a little beaten down.

Get out your pom-poms and cheer your new cheer. We say: "I can do it! I value myself enough to make time in my busy schedule to exercise. I have the ability to just say no to the excess food that is always knocking at my mind or in my eyes' view. My worth is of importance and I will not think otherwise."

"My health and wellness are essential and I won't minimize that fact. I feel great after an awesome workout, and the choice to do it is never regretted. Good food choices are delicious and doing awesome things inside my body, whether I see that truth or not. My mind is crisp, sharp, and alert with exercise a part of my daily life, and I refuse to lay down to sedentary days and sit in a lethargic and sluggish state of mind."

"The ballgame is not over and it's never ever too late to just do it. I will think positive thoughts about myself and will refuse to nitpick myself to death to keep from reaching my full potential."

I challenge you to cheer this pep talk cheer as many times as you need to.

Are You in a Funk?
Day 205

Emotions, emotions and more emotions - everybody has them. No one is exempt from them. Some have more extreme highs and lows than others, but we all have the God-given ability to feel. Often, when it's time to exercise, our emotions take a front seat. Thoughts magnify, such as: I don't feel very good; I'm tired; I'm not seeing any results; I've got too much to do; this is a waste of my time; I'm bored; I feel ginormous; I'm not losing any weight.

I call these feelings an emotional funk. I want to address these emotions. If we don't address these feelings, we soon follow them right out the gym door, never to return. I have a conversation with myself when I'm feeling low. It goes something like this: "I'm tired and bored; I'm exercising anyway," or "I feel ginormous; I'm exercising anyway." We must come up with words to counteract the emotions that lead us toward a funk.

From a very young age, I got a hold of a false reality about myself. I believed, and still to this day fight, these words: "I'm fat, white, and ugly." Daily, I thought this of myself. You may be laughing to yourself. It's silly, BUT these three words led me down a road of eating and exercise disorders. These three little words have plagued me for as long as I can remember. I still have to counteract them most days.

It's a must to come up with an antidote against your funk. Stay aware of what you are thinking. My antidote, "I'm exercising anyway," has kept my funk at bay all of my life. Exercise has leveled out unwanted emotions. It's been my therapy. You DO feel better after exercise. I encourage you to hang on; the funk passes.

Perfection vs. Balance and Moderation
Day 206

We all desire a good bill of health. But the pursuit of good health and wellness, as we know, is driven by a desire from deep within us. A question that is a must to get straight in our minds is this; is your desire propelled by the pursuit of perfection or by the pursuit of balance and moderation?

The pursuit of perfection will have you jumping from one program to another; looking at one fitness magazine model after another and wondering how do I attain that look; how do I get from where I am to where they are? This way of pursuit does not work. I know this firsthand, because for years I based my career in the health and wellness industry in pursuit of perfection. Perfection is unattainable for many reasons. For instance, we all possess a natural critical perception of ourselves. We're never satisfied and are imperfect, which makes the realization of the "perfection" goal unachievable.

Perfection is not attainable. I can't say it enough. If we continue striving for perfection, a defeatist attitude will cause us to never want to try again. After learning the hard way, I challenge you to not go after something that can never be attained.

The real key to health and wellness is balance and moderation. Balance and moderation is everything perfection is not. I encourage you to release yourself from the burden of trying to seek perfection. Set goals that are attainable, goals that are simple and based on balance and moderation. Movement of any sort. Movement is underrated. Walking in the park, riding bikes, or hiking all are simple but do your body wonders. Take time to reassess your health and wellness journey. Are you in balance? Is your approach moderate? Constant evaluation is key.

Fabulous at Any Age
Day 207

 Facing a new decade of life can seem a little daunting.

Karen was facing her fifties with a determination to be different. I'm proud to say she hit this new decade of years head-on and here's her story:

"About 6 months ago I decided to work out. I said I would get serious when I turned 50, but here I was at 51 and still not doing it. Anyway - I committed to a company fitness class and started telling the trainer that I'd see her in the next one (my word is my word and the only way I could think to keep the momentum going was to promise to be in class). It took about 4 months for the exercise high to kick in, but when it finally did I started feeling great (both physically and mentally). I've lost a few pounds and firmed up some muscles, but the greatest reward has been how much better I feel. I have more energy than I've had in a very long time. Thank you to my company for giving me this opportunity. It is truly a blessing in my life."

Karen's commitment to exercise has resulted in a phenomenal change in her body composition. Initially, Karen dreaded exercise; now she anticipates it and it shows! She is looking great in her 50's and is a wonderful example that life isn't over at 50.

I want to encourage you to look at each new year and each new day as an opportunity to continue to learn and improve your life. Exercising on a regular basis will allow you to remain mobile, flexible, independent, and fabulous as your life goes on.

Truth or Dare
Day 208

What happens when you quit something? We can all testify to quitting. Quitting usually leaves you feeing guilty, thinking about all the what ifs and the thought that you should've hung in there. If you're thinking of quitting fitness, I have a question for you. What would happen if you didn't give up? That reminds me of the game "Truth or Dare."

The Truth is if you don't give up you'll reap a plentiful harvest. I Dare you to find out.

Let's play the game.

Truth: You're more productive when you're active, having increased energy from endorphins.

Truth: Regular exercise can prevent illness.

Truth: Aerobic exercise is linked to a better memory.

Truth: People who don't regularly exercise may lose up to 80% of their muscle strength by age 65.

Truth: Your heart is the hardest working muscle in your body. It beats approximately 100,000 times per day, pumping almost 2,000 gallons of blood.

Truth: During physical activity, you breathe harder to keep oxygen in your blood at appropriate levels.

Truth: Fat and muscle are completely different types of tissue. Muscle cannot turn into fat and vice versa.

Now, the most important part of the game is I DARE you to take a lifetime to find out what exactly does happen if you never give up. You may fall, but falling and quitting are two different things. Have no fear, because you will rise again. Proverbs 24:16 says, "The righteous man may suffer adversity and stumble seven times, but they will continue to rise over and over again."

When good advice is in "The Word," I always get excited. I leave you with this challenge: Dare to never give up! On your mark ... get set ... GO.

Small Changes Make Big Differences
Day 209

rest day

Bodies are constantly changing, from our skin cells down to the very core of our bones. We're either growing bigger, smaller, or we're working our bodies hard to simply maintain through this change. We should never take our health for granted. It's a blessing to wake up to another day healthy.

A great way to jumpstart your bodies as they rapidly change is to add something good and omit something not so good. This even applies to maintaining our body weight and muscle mass. Whether you need to lose, gain, or maintain weight, your body is going through its cycle of constant change.

Small decisions of making good health choices can leave you with a discovery of small blessings that can become big blessings. A new healthy habit can increase your energy levels, making you able to get more done in your day. With this new vigor, you'll experience a sense of great accomplishment.

I challenge you to embrace making small healthy choices. I guarantee you'll be amazed at what you discover about yourself when you make a few small changes.

One of my very own clients told me how she had been to a birthday party that was serving two of her favorites, M&M's and German chocolate cake. Even though she was faced with some of her favorite desserts, she made the decision not to indulge. With this small decision of saying no thank you, she left the party with a great sense of accomplishment.

A sense of accomplishment is sometimes just as rewarding as losing weight. With a sense of accomplishment comes confidence in yourself. Change for better is possible.

Seize a Fitness Moment
Day 210

rest day We must seize opportunities to be all we can be. Too often we sell ourselves short of our full potential. This is especially true when it comes to fitness. Our individual bodies are specifically made to move and eat a certain amount daily; however, our flesh is weak.

There's an optimal choice each day brings. The question, "Am I ready to seize all the physical opportunities I can today?" must be asked daily. Before you let the "yeah, but…" excuses steal your day, consider the physical desires you have and set goals for yourself.

Recognize things that hold you back, push them out of the way, and get on with being proactive. Act first – second-guess yourself later. You can do it! Believe in yourself; all things are possible. What are you waiting for? Only you can do it for you. Only you can make it happen.

For example: Move for ten continual minutes. Do my video at the same allotted time each day. I know you want to feel better. I know you want to look better. These small goals will achieve both of these normal desires. Don't waste one more day.

I challenge you to start by taking time to make one very small do-able goal today. I also encourage you to get one good meal under your belt. Our daily race should be to not put off until tomorrow what we can accomplish today.

Hebrews 12:1 (NIV) "Therefore, since we are surrounded by such a great cloud of witnesses, let us throw off everything that hinders and the sin that so easily entangles, and let us run with perseverance the race marked out for us."

Seize your fitness moment today.

Sickness CANNOT Fully Manifest!
Day 211

If you're constantly pursuing better health and wellness, sickness may try to come knocking at your door, but it's not allowed to stay. If you're wondering what in the world I'm talking about, let me share. There are health problems associated with certain lifestyle choices, especially lack of exercise.

Let's review the basics of a healthy lifestyle:

Cardiorespiratory Exercise: Adults should get at least 150 minutes of moderate-intensity exercise per week. Exercise can be met through 30 to 60 minutes of moderate-intensity exercise five days per week or 20 to 60 minutes of vigorous-intensity exercise three days per week.

Resistance Exercise: Adults should train each major muscle group two or three days each week using a variety of exercises and equipment. Very light or light intensity is best for older individuals or previously sedentary adults just starting to exercise. Two to four sets of each exercise, with anywhere between eight and 20 repetitions, will help adults improve strength and power.

Flexibility Exercise: Adults should do flexibility exercises at least two or three days each week to improve range of motion. Each stretch should be held for 10 to 30 seconds, to the point of tightness or slight discomfort.

Functional Fitness Training Exercises: Should be done two or three days per week. Exercises should involve motor skills (balance, agility, coordination, and gait), proprioceptive exercise training, and multifaceted activities (yoga) to improve physical function and prevent falls in older adults.

These reminders in your pursuit to better health have everything to do with keeping sickness at bay. I'm not denying people get sick, but a healthy body has no time for sickness to stick around. I don't know about you, but that's good news to me. Let's go forward together and stay on the HEALTHY TRAIN.

Winning Strategies
Day 212

If you've been exercising for any length of time, you've probably already figured out that winning at weight loss is about making long-lasting, life-altering change. Just like any sport or skill, you might start out a little rocky because learning the strategies takes practice.

Here are some winning strategies to practice to help you stay successful:

Your journey is a battle. Your mind must be in the game. Whether you're focusing on your diet or you're working out hard, the commitment to long-term weight loss takes the mindset and mental stamina of a champion.

Winners take breaks and time outs. When you first set out to shed pounds, it's easy to overdo it. Take a diet timeout to enjoy a slice of cake at a friend's birthday party. Schedule a relaxing soak in the tub on your day off from the gym.

You've gotta have fun. In order to win, you need to make it fun. What do parents tell their kids the first time they try a new game or sport? "It isn't about whether you win or lose, just have fun." The same advice applies to weight loss. Worrying too much about your waistline can actually cause you to engage in stress eating or become too depressed to work out.

Whether you've discovered a new dog park near home, convinced a coworker to join you in making healthier food choices at lunch, or found new ways to burn calories, have fun. I'll bet while stepping out to experiment with ways to stay healthy, some great experiences will come your way.

A healthy lifestyle is pretty much cut and dry; you're either on or off. I challenge you to ask yourself if you're winning at your health or losing. It's never too late to choose to win!

Does Exercise Affect Your Hormones?
Day 213

As your personal trainer, the guidelines for what I'm able to discuss are limited. Hormones are very specific in what they can do. When an individual exercises, there are many different physical adaptations the body must go through.

First, it's good to know hormones are released into your bloodstream. Hormones will only act at specific sites, known as receptors, within your body. Once a hormone has bonded to a receptor on a cell, it can send messages to the cell and tell it (and effectively the body as a whole) to perform a specific function.

Example: hormones act like managers who tell their employees what to do. Just like a manager has a specific role in an employee's life, hormones are also specific in what they can tell the body to do. Therefore, one (or possibly a few) bodily functions or adaptations to exercise can be regulated by specific hormones.

Testosterone has been considered the holy grail of muscle building. Testosterone blood serum levels can be increased during heavy strength and weight training. The hormone promotes protein synthesis.

Testosterone will also support and increase production of new red blood cells, which leads to an increased ability to utilize oxygen more effectively. It also leads to more efficient usage of glucose, which leads to less difficulty when performing strenuous exercise. This is why it is often abused by athletes in an attempt to enhance performance.

Growth Hormone is a chain of 191 amino acids. These amino acids, when grouped together, can instruct the body to perform protein synthesis and cell transport. What's good to know is Growth Hormone is secreted in response to exercise.

Who knew hormones can be affected by exercise? If you feel like your hormones are out of sorts, consult your physician.

We Mustn't Forget the Basics
Day 214

Each day my heart's desire is to bring you a "wowsie truth" about fitness. As I was thinking about what to share today, I thought about reminding you to keep the basics as the foundation, then build from there. I encourage you to learn all about the next fad. Do the latest and greatest new thing, just don't stop growing. As you move forward in seeking out these fun, new, exciting things health and wellness has to offer, don't forget to always build on the basics, or you will find yourself not making progress.

There are no short term answers. Continue to commit for the long term. Short-term anything won't last. You can apply your new latest and greatest routine, like added intensity, to your basic fitness.

If you're adding the new fad diet to your basic nutrition, make sure you progress SLOWLY. Don't leave behind your basic lean meats, vegetables, and fruits. There's no trick to eating properly. Once again, it's the slow progress made day after day, week after week, month after month, and year after year that produces a fit, healthy body.

But, these fads could be your answers to breaking fitness plateaus. When finding you're not making much progress, you can use what you've learned from a new fad to break your fitness plateau. Your health and wellness journey is endless. Trying all you can keeps things vibrant and moving successfully forward.

You should embrace this journey with excitement, determination, and seriousness. You WILL choose to keep basic fitness part of your plan. This will ensure you to be the best you can be. You're worth it. Just ask your loved ones around you. They'd agree, you're SPECIAL and worth the fight.

Lean or Bulky
Day 215

Ladies, have you ever wanted to have skinny legs when instead you look down at two nicely plump ones? Or you might have skinny legs and want muscular ones? Men, have you ever wanted a nice muscular chest and biceps, but instead look in the mirror at a not-so-muscular one? Or you may have too much upper body mass and would be happy to have lean washboard abs in front?

I'm pretty sure we all want a certain physical attribute that we simply don't have the genetics to ever have. The hard truth is, we must consider our body type as we seek better health. According to the American College of Sports Medicine, it's largely a myth that weightlifting causes women to bulk up.

It is true, however, that the tendency to develop bulky or lean muscles varies widely from one person to the next. While the male hormone, testosterone, does contribute to muscle growth, body type is just as important a factor in how your body responds to strength training.

If you have a muscular mesomorph body type, you'll quickly take on more muscle mass. If you're a more voluptuous endomorph, you'll typically lose weight before you see notable growth in muscle. Slim ectomorphs are unlikely to ever develop bulky muscles, even as they become stronger. Strength training is good for all body types but will always produce different exterior results.

Whatever body type category you find yourself in, do strength training at least twice per week, but never train the same muscles two days in a row. Whatever your heart's desire may be, first embrace who God made you to be. You're beautiful/handsome and uniquely made!! Then set some realistic goals, seek a plan, and go for it. YOU CAN DO IT.

Unexpected Happenstance
Day 216

rest day   Did you know there are four major roadblocks that hit us starting in the eighth month every year? First, there's back to school in August or September. Second, there's the time change in October. Third, there's the cold weather settling in late November. Fourth, there's the holiday season in November and December. If you can hang on to some sort of normality beginning in August and not let go until the New Year, then you have a chance to make it through with flying colors.

I hope you're making it through with flying colors this season, but chances are you'll fight for a sense of normality at some point in time. I'd like to discuss the unexpected happenstances that still hit even when you feel you're doing all you can to stay afloat. Unexpected happenstances usually occur right smack dab in the center of already interrupted schedules and other mishaps life throws at you.

Here are some things you can use when you're faced with unexpected happenstance:

- Do what you can. Don't focus on what you can't do.
- If you have a quick weight gain or weight loss, know that your body likes a certain weight and will fight to stay there.
- Don't allow an event to get you out of the game. Your health is not optional; it's a necessity .
- Don't allow all the strikes against you to make you throw in the towel and quit.

I challenge you to keep exercise a routine part of life. No joke. Whatever roadblocks or unexpected happenstances come your way, keep fitness a priority.

Colon Facts
Day 217

rest day

Have you ever wondered how often you should visit the bathroom? Bathroom visits will vary from person to person. Everybody is different, and there is no set "normal" time when it comes to passing stools.

But, research does state the normal range spans from three times a day to once every three days. There is even a healthy shape of your stool. Some medical experts say the ideal stool shape should hold together and take roughly the form of an "S." This truth is based on the fact that the colon and intestines are long and thin, so the ideal stool should adopt a similar shape.

An individual's age, gender, weight, current exercise routine, health issues, and even hormones can affect digestion/metabolism, which in turn affects bathroom visits.

Take age as an example. First, your metabolism will slow down a little, which could decrease the number of times you visit the bathroom in a day. People also become more prone to constipation as they age. This may be a result of medication, trouble moving around, or simply not getting enough water or fiber in the diet.

Researchers have proven that a few stretches in the morning along with a diet rich in fiber and an increased intake of water should help in many cases! If these things don't help, you might want to check with your physician.

I had to take my daughter to the emergency room not too long ago, as she was doubled over in stomach pain. Her outcome was a blessing; nothing serious. The doctor told me that 85% of emergency visits are stomach related.

I encourage you to put digestion, bladder, and colon health on your radar. Things like these should be a priority! Remember, we only have one go-round.

HIIT vs Metabolic Training
Day 218

High Intensity Interval Training (HIIT) and Metabolic Training are two methods of exercise. I'd like to talk about their differences.

HIIT is a style of working out that alternates between segments of low intensity and very high intensity using cardiovascular exercises. HIIT uses exercises like jogging, sprinting, and rowing.

Metabolic training emphasizes more resistance training protocols like kettle bell squats with overhead presses, or dumbbell side lunges followed by side rows. It requires times of high intensity with times of lower intensity while adjusting weights.

The lines between these two methods are blurry. One could argue that a sprint workout is metabolically intense just as a weighted metabolic workout is cardiovascularly intense.

Everyone's fitness should be founded on the fundamentals of fitness. Every individual's exercise program should include: (1) strength, (2) cardio, and (3) flexibility. Then a HIIT or metabolic training method would be a great variation to add to your foundation.

These methods are great ways to push and compete with yourself. They can be used as a measuring tool for growth based on your last HIIT record times or metabolic training weight increases. Keep a journal so you can stay encouraged.

I challenge you to try both methods. HIIT being based on cardiovascular blasts and metabolic training being more of a resistance training protocol are both a win-win to add to your workouts. I recommend a little bit of both. Personally, due to a lot of overuse injuries, I lean more toward the metabolic training because I can get more benefit out of the resistance intensity and stay low impact.

The design of both HIIT and metabolic training formats gives your metabolism a jolt. They leave your metabolic rate high for the rest of the day. Add some spice to your fitness foundation and try one.

Don't Judge a Book by Its Cover
Day 219

Health and wellness is an individual walk. Whether you're short or wide, tall or thin, we all have challenges. All too often, we have a tendency to pay less attention to the story of the people who we view as thin.

I encourage you to never judge a book by its cover of others needs not being as real as yours and mine.

Here is a testimony of a tall, thin, beautiful client of mine:

"When I started class I was a size 14 and weighed 148 pounds at the first weigh-in. I had been very frustrated with the weight I gained during my second pregnancy and did not have luck with keeping weight off after I had the baby. I would lose a few and gain a few back and yo-yoed like that for several months.

I really thought with getting older the weight was simply not going to come off (I weighed 125 before I learned I was pregnant and gained 50 pounds through the end of pregnancy). After starting the program in August, I have lost 19 pounds (last weigh in I was at 129 pounds) and am now a size 8.

I believe the weekly classes and accountability have kept me on track and focused on my goal, which was to return to my pre-pregnancy weight; I have about 4 pounds to go!!! I feel better physically and mentally than I have in years and am grateful to the company for including me in this program. It's been key in helping me to attain my fitness goals!"

Let's not judge others. I want to encourage you to be open to learning about the cry of others. The very struggles they have might be just what you need for your health and wellness success.

Facing Inevitable Changes
Day 220

There are three things in life that are bound to change: life, weather, and your body. You may have a little insight into when some changes may happen, but you can't predict them all with any real certainty. In pursuing a life of health and wellness, it's the "changes" that will keep us on our toes.

Just as you watch the rapid changes in your child's body, you can be rest assured your body is changing as well. Don't hate your body for it, it's just doing what it's designed to do. Even if you find you're putting on a little too much weight, losing too much weight, or feeling some new aches and pains, don't see these as signs to stop exercising.

Instead, look at these signs as an opportunity to evaluate where you are. Maybe you need to adjust your old standard routine or try something new. Be aware, old habits are sometimes hard to break. Don't stop trying to find new ways. Any time spent on health and wellness is a positive investment. Exercise could be the very thing that is keeping you sane and getting you through whatever season you may be facing in life right now.

If you're fit and doing well, keep up the great work. If the years are slipping by and you've found yourself sedentary, then hop on board today starting with one minor choice to get back into exercising or healthy eating. Good choices always reap results.

If your life is one big change, it's okay. There's still some sunlight left to make a small good choice. Someone told me years ago, "Don't put off until tomorrow what you can do today." Let's take change by the horns and get moving. You'll be glad you did.

Intensity is Here to Stay
Day 221

I just completed my continuing education class this weekend. I chose HIIT training because it's all the craze right now. I'd like to share some important things I learned about intensity.

Intensity plays a big role in our results. This is why it's all the craze, but you must realize it takes a delicate balance.

When you enter a phase of your workout that's intense, you should really be listening to your body's response. There's a fine line of intensity where you can push yourself too hard or not hard enough.

Here are two basic ways to make intensity work for you.

Measure your intensity based on how you feel. This is called Perceived Exertion Scale. It's intensity based on a subjective measure of how hard physical activity "feels" during your workout. It's measured by numbers; one being the easiest and ten being the hardest.

The second measure is based on heart rate. Your heart rate offers a more objective look at exercise intensity. In this world of technology, heart rates can easily be monitored by a plethora of fitness watches you can purchase. The higher your heart rate is during physical activity, the higher the intensity and vice-versa.

Once you understand your exercise intensity, you can get really creative. You can choose your exercise intensity by adding aerobic activity to strength training. You can get creative by pairing free weights, weight machines, or even activities that use your own body weight.

You must remember balance is important. Overdoing it at 100% intensity all the time can increase your risk of soreness, injury, and burnout. On the flip side, if you never explore your own personal intensity, you're selling yourself short. I hope you'll explore new heights and discover new wisdom to keep you in this beautiful game of fitness.

Something Effective You Can Do at Home
Day 222

A question I'm frequently asked: "What exercises can I do at home?" When you're in the gym, you have all the latest equipment right at your fingertips. I love the gym, but unfortunately it's not always feasible to get there.

You can still be productive at home without having everything that the gym offers. What's the solution? Your own body weight! Two very effective fitness "tools" readily available at all times are your bodyweight and gravity!

These two elements allow you to exercise anywhere, anytime. Here are some safe, effective, and challenging bodyweight exercises you can do at home.

Hand Dance Push Up. How to: Get into a push up position. Perform a push up, followed by moving your right hand/right foot only, outwards. Perform another push up, then bring your right arm and leg back in. Repeat on left side. 15-20 repetitions (3 times)

Upper Body Jack Squat. How to: Begin by standing up, arms overhead and feet a comfortable distance apart for squatting. As you drop down into the squat, drop your arms out and down to the side (as you would with your arms when performing a jumping jack). As you rise from the bottom of the squat, lift your arms out to the side and up so that when you return to the standing position, your arms are once again overhead. 15-20 repetitions (3 times)

Bird Dog on the Bench. How to: Begin with both hands and the right knee on a bench or chair. Lift your left leg out to the side then back down with your toes gently resting on the floor. Repeat with the opposite arm/leg combination.15-20 repetitions (3 times)

Body weight exercises are good for everyone. Fortunately, no equipment is required. I challenge you to try this routine.

Continual Quest for Change
Day 223

rest day Life is busy for most of us, and finding time for a workout can be challenging. When you do find time, you want to make sure you're getting the most "bang for your buck," being as efficient as possible with your workout program. Making small changes to your current routine can do more than you think.

Change can increase your calorie burn, improve your fitness level, and make your health-related goals even more attainable. I'd like to share a couple of ideas on how to change things up.

Cardiovascular ideas:

Treadmill exerciser? Try a stationary bike. Stationary biking can be a great workout that's low-impact and easy on your joints. Spinning classes are a good option for staying focused and pushing yourself just as hard as a good run.

Walking exerciser? Try Interval Walking. Starting with a consistent pace and slowly building up your distance and speed is a great way to challenge yourself and improve your fitness level.

Resistance Training ideas:

Is your "go to" crunches? Try planks. The traditional crunch only targets your upper abdominal area. Planks not only strengthen all of your abdominal muscles, but also your shoulders and hips.

High reps, low weight exerciser? Try low reps, high weight. When it comes to strength training, "high reps, low weight" is a popular recommendation. A high rep, low weight option can be 100 squats or lunges, for example. It's time to find a way to increase the intensity (up weight) and decrease the number of reps (6-8).

I encourage you to be on a continual quest for change. Changing your workout routine regularly can also help avoid both fitness and weight-loss plateaus. Don't be afraid to try something new. You never know what goals are waiting to be achieved. You can do fitness.

The Unwanted
Day 224

Numerous times over the years, I've thought about how we want that quick fix when it comes to exercise. Usually a special event or vacation plan will push us to the gym for that miracle fix. Truth be told, what we really need is a mindset change in the way we think about our overall health and wellness. Fitness isn't a quick destination; it's a lifelong journey.

Here is a good little jingle to remember, "Every single day, we must chip away all the unwanted that wants to stay." Now, that's a truth to live by. Exercise is an adventure that needs to be done most days of the week all year long.

This jingle also applies to other unwanted areas of our lives that cause us to struggle, become frustrated, or disappoint us. Examples of these unwanted conditions include weight gain or loss, bad skin, emotional issues, stress, rehab from an injury or surgery, problematic job or relationships, and the list goes on.

When it comes to dealing with our unwanted, there are two ways to handle them.

One is to ignore the falsehood of unwanted:
1. I'm too fat to do that exercise. Ignore!
2. I can't walk 5 miles. Ignore!
3. I've never been fit. Ignore!
4. Health and wellness is impossible for me. Ignore!

Two is to address the unwanted with exercise:
1. Stress
2. Pandemic 30-pound weight gain
3. Depression
4. Hopelessness (Seek professional help, too. There is no shame in getting help.)

Now that you know what needs to be ignored or dealt with, I pray you will begin to recognize and ignore the lies, deal with your excuses and face the issues at hand, and deal with those issues you have the power to change. You can do this!

Do I Need to Eat More
on Cardio/Weightlifting Days?
Day 225

YES! You do need more calories on weightlifting/cardiovascular training days. You can look at it like this: if you were going on a long trip, would you need more gas? Of course! It's a given that you're going to have to stop and fill up several times to get to your final destination. Your body is the same way.

If you wake up earlier, or workout harder, it's guaranteed that you'll need to consume more calories that day. "How many calories do I need," you ask? Everyone wants to know how much food is normal to consume.

Within my personal training guidelines, I'm able to recommend 65% carbohydrates, 15% proteins, and 20% fats. The total amount of calories from these three sources will vary based on activity performance. A registered dietitian can prescribe the exact amount of calories you'll need on rest days as well as active days. Starting your day with a plan will always help you keep your portion sizes and caloric intake in check.

I'd like to share some foods that are considered healthy carbohydrates, proteins, and fats that you can eat more of on your active days.

Healthy carbohydrates to consume on workout days are sweet potatoes, yogurts, cottage cheese, whole grains (pastas/quinoa/rices), and fruits/vegetables.

Healthy proteins to consume on workout days are eggs, chicken/lean beef/fish, milk, and protein powder drinks.

Healthy fats to consume on workout days are avocado, peanut butter/almond butter, olive oils, and nuts.

You now have some basic foods to choose from. The biggest tip for today is to listen to your body's queues for its need for food. Whatever your hunger signs may be, feed it good fuel and more when needed. We all need a specific plan.

Thoughts ... Thoughts ... and More Thoughts
Day 226

Have you ever heard someone say, "Be careful what you ponder on because your actions will surely follow?" It's a must to reverse wrong thinking into positive self-talk. I'd like to give you some thinking tools that will help you stay focused and in the game of fitness. Here are a few positive thinking tools that lead to being the best YOU.

I challenge you to tell yourself these truths:

Exercise does matter TODAY. You have only one today. If you put off the good you can do for yourself today, it could lead to inconsistency. Being unaware of the negative pull can eventually drown you. So, TODAY does matter...EXERCISE.

You DO have time to EXERCISE. Life is busy for all of us. Plan out when and where you'll fit in your workout. Remember, your health and wellness is just as important as your paycheck.

Just do it. Sure, you might have dreaded thoughts at the beginning of your workout. But the beautiful truth is you never ever regret making the choice to exercise. When you complete a workout, never ever do you say, "I wish I hadn't exercised today." Every single time you just do it, you'll feel a sense of accomplishment. You'll feel better than you did before your workout.

Remember, what you think or ponder on soon turns into action. I encourage you to purposely think about how you WILL execute your daily fitness regimen and good nutrition choices, no matter what the day brings you.

You'll never regret the choices that produce better health. Exercise, anyone? Clean eating, anyone? Of course. Just remember it's possible and it's never ever too late. You can do it.

Do the Types of Calories Eaten Matter?
Day 227

I saw an ad on social media that had a McDonald's hamburger in one hand and a protein bar in the other. The point of the ad was that the hamburger was 300 calories and the protein bar was 360 calories, suggesting the hamburger was the better option.

Which one do you think is better? The protein bar. Yes, it's higher in calories. Sure, you do need to be aware of your total caloric intake, but the type of calories really do matter. When you're burning calories, a calorie burned is a calorie burned, but how your body responds to each "calorie" is not the same.

If you eat fried food all day then want to perform well for an athletic event, the fried food diet will most likely hinder your performance. My daughter bought bad gas not too long ago. Her car was hissing and popping and carrying on. We thought we had some serious problems. We made an appointment with the car dealership, but the next day on the radio we heard the news report of bad gas in the area.

We soon discovered that her car simply had bad gas. When she filled up with good gas, all the hissing and carrying on stopped. The same goes for your body. Good fats, lean meats, fruits, and vegetables are great fuel to make your body feel and perform fantastically.

It's a must for all of us to weigh out the pros and cons of our food choices. It really does matter what kind of calories you consume. One of my dad's favorite sayings when I was growing up was, "You can only eat an elephant one bite at a time." We all have "elephants" to conquer. So simply become aware of the type of calories you eat.

A Little Goes a Long Way
Day 228

You've been given a twenty-four hour day, and your job usually takes up most of the day. A blessing is it only takes about 20-60 minutes out of a twenty-four hour period to become fit. A little exercise can go a long way.

People have more energy at different times of the day. Either people love to exercise in the morning or they prefer evenings. Believe it or not, some people like neither and that's okay, too.

Let's look at the benefits of morning, evening, or lunchtime workouts to inspire you.

Benefits of Morning Exercise:

• Boosts your metabolism. You can burn 20% more calories consumed at breakfast if you exercise before eating.

• Helps you stay more active all day long. It's like a natural caffeine boost.

• Helps you get a better night's sleep.

• Boosts your immune system to better fight off sickness.

• Fewer distractions makes for a better workout and helps you focus the rest of the day.

Benefits of Evening Exercise:

• Relieves your body tension.

• Warm-ups are done through your day's activities.

• Workouts can be longer.

• Helps you sleep more deeply.

• Ends your day in a great way and sets you up for an incredible day tomorrow.

Benefits of Midday Exercise:

• Boosts your mood and energy levels.

• Improves your problem-solving skills.

• Creates more free time before and after work.

• Reduces work stress.

• Saves money because you exercise instead of buying lunch.

Some of these may seem a bit silly, but sometimes motivation is really that simple. What do you say? Find some small, allotted time period in your day and run with it. You won't regret it. A little time set aside to exercise goes a long, long way.

243

Appetite vs Hunger
Day 229

People eat for two reasons: they are either hungry or their appetite is speaking to them. Hunger and appetite are not synonymous. They are entirely different entities.

Hunger is the need for food. Every time you eat, your pancreas secretes insulin, which is a hormone that enables you to transform the food you eat into glucose. Thus, when the glucose circulating in your blood declines, your body is signaled with thoughts of food as your brain picks up on the physical reaction in your stomach. These work together to signal you to eat.

Appetite, however, is the desire for food. It is the basis for the familiar saying, "Your eyes are bigger than your stomach." It is a sensory or psychological reaction when something looks good or smells good to you which stimulates an involuntary physiological response such as salivation and stomach contractions.

Let's look at an example. You decide to have hot dogs for lunch. If you are hungry, you will eat only one hot dog. After that, your appetite may lead you to eat two more hot dogs because they look appealing or tasted good.

I'm very appetite-driven myself. So I always do a test run to determine if I'm hungry or if it's my appetite. I ask myself, "Could I eat spinach, sweet potato, and chicken?" If I say, "Yes," then I am hungry. If I tell myself, "No, I'm in the mood for something sweet," then I'm not hungry.

Before you pack on the calories, I challenge you to first ask yourself the following question. "Am I hungry or is this my appetite speaking?" With practice, you will learn to recognize the difference between hunger and appetite in your own body, and then you can better eat for fitness.

An Unchanging Truth
Day 230

rest day The only way to be successful in weight loss is to burn more calories than you consume. One pound of fat is equivalent to 3.500 calories. That's an unchanging truth. We are all unique and metabolize calories differently, but we still have to burn off more than we consume.

Let's do some simple math and biology to better explain our bodies. Math first. Let's take a 150-pound woman who drinks one less cup of reduced-fat milk per day. She will lose more than 104 pounds over the next ten years. That is 365,000 calories divided by 3,500 calories per pound of fat which equals 104 pounds of fat.

These amazing results are produced by cutting a measly 100 calories through eliminating one cup of reduced-fat milk per day. Obviously, our bodies are not black and white like math. Our bodies are really biology projects in progress. We need the mathematical equations because it's factual information that best helps lead and guide us toward better health.

Now for biology class. The biology of your body can't be ignored. Sicknesses, certain diseases, medications, and differing rates of metabolism can affect the black-and-white mathematical equation of your body. Your doctor can give you specific information about how your body works.

One thing we all have in common within our biological makeup is food is the tool needed for fat loss and weight loss. Food used in the right way will keep your metabolic rate up and keep it highly functional. It's up to us to learn about our biological makeup and seek the right foods and times to eat to operate at peak efficiency.

I challenge you to learn your unique body and handle your unchanging truth (3,500 calories will always equal a pound of fat) with care.

Delete the Defeat
Day 231

I'd like to share two things pertaining to deleting unwanted, false information.

First, at a wonderful little church revival, they had a 'Love Feast' that consisted of a gathering of people sharing how their lives had been the previous year. One lady (80 years old) stood up and shared, from her heart, about having a critical/judgmental spirit. She shared how she battles thinking in a negative way of people and was struggling how not to be so hard on them. She went on to say she has learned to turn her thoughts into a prayer for the person that she is thinking negatively toward.

Second, I'm learning how to delete critical/judgmental thoughts about myself. Our minds are like computers in need of reprogramming. We need to learn how to hit the delete button. When negative, discouraging thoughts are trying to contaminate your software, hit delete before those thoughts start affecting how you live.

These are some defeating thoughts:

I'm fat; I'll always be overweight…DELETE.

I can't do that; I'm too young…DELETE.

I can't begin something new; I'm too old…DELETE.

I've always been unattractive; I'll never meet the people I'm supposed to meet…DELETE.

I'm not good enough…DELETE.

I'm dumb; I've always been a C student; I'm not college material…DELETE.

I don't have what it takes…DELETE.

I've seen my best day; it's only going downhill from here…DELETE.

I'll never recover from my recent surgery; I might as well quit…DELETE.

I'll never break this addiction; I might as well throw in the towel…DELETE.

You might laugh at some of those thoughts because you can't relate, but thoughts can be dangerous. Your very thoughts become action.

I challenge you to try to think positively and just see if your life gets better.

The Simplicity of Decision
Day 232

Today, I'd like to be short and simple. One thing that never gets old in the fitness industry is a success story. I had the honor of remeasuring a client and celebrating her results. She lost a considerable amount of scale weight and 12 inches in overall body measurements. I walked away so inspired.

She put in the hard work and reaped the benefits. It got me thinking about how we all decide to make a simple decision for change one ordinary day. At that particular moment, our minds are filled with hope of what this simple decision will bring: you'll lose weight, you'll be stronger, you'll have more endurance, you'll look better, you'll feel better, etc., and then you take action to make that change.

As I began to ask my precious client about her success, she shared with me that she happened to try a particular diet her friend recommended, and within one week she lost 6 pounds. To her surprise, she continued eating that new way in hopes to lose more. She then made another simple decision to begin an exercise regime slowly and optimistically within her body limitations.

She found a class she enjoyed and kept at it until she grew in strength and stamina. She's still growing stronger today. I remember passing through the gym when her class was over, and she was still there on the floor doing her extra stretches for her certain body limitations. By golly, she was there, putting in the extra time and pushing through. What an encouraging sight to see!

Let's make the simple decision to push through on those days where we can't seem to find the benefit. Let's stay positive because the decision to make one simple change ALWAYS produces results.

Exercise is a Mental Battle
Day 233

Face it, some days we dread exercising. The danger lies in if we focus on the notion for too long, it could easily lead to inconsistency. Inconsistency in exercise is a silent killer. We must exercise most days a week; however, being unaware of the pull of not wanting to can eventually drown us.

Before we know it, we haven't exercised in a month. For example, a beginner exerciser who is fresh into the habit of exercising will have to battle thoughts of dread soon. To counteract those defeating thoughts, a couple simple steps can help. The night before, you can lay out your exercise clothes, so when your morning alarm goes off, there's little to no thought about not exercising.

Some days there needs to be a set time to exercise so it doesn't interfere with the rest of your day. Your exercise time can be ruined by thinking about the thousand other things that need to get done. When your uninterrupted exercise time is completed and out of the way, you can carry out your daily tasks with an extra vigor you wouldn't have if you skipped exercising.

Mentally telling yourself no regrets. After a workout, you never say, "I wish I hadn't exercised today." Every time you do it, the benefits always remind you why you love exercise.

The mental battle will always be a reckoning force to deal with. Don't give into it. Continue to make room in your day to exercise. It's in your best interest and the best interest of those around you.

You'll never regret the choice. Exercise is a battle. I encourage you to believe it's possible to win daily. So what do you say? Exercise, anyone? Of course, you would love to exercise!

Grace to the Diehard Exerciser
Day 234

Have you ever heard somebody say, "You're addicted to exercise?" This is a constructive addiction, but as with anything extreme, there's a downside. I'd like to talk to the diehard exerciser today.

I remember when I was pregnant the first question I asked my doctor was, "How soon after delivery can I exercise?" Right after giving birth is the most valid time to not work out. It's typically recommended that you wait six weeks post-delivery before you begin workouts again. This rule is even longer if you've had a C-section. Heed your doctor's advice. Enjoy your newborn. Don't rush back into fitness until your body feels ready to take it on. There will be plenty of time to work out once you've recovered.

If you've been set back for reasons out of your control, this is a great time to discover new, less strenuous exercises like bike riding, rowing, or a low-impact exercise class. Being stubborn by doing what you've always done and not listening to your body's needs will set you back even more. Give yourself grace. Work with your doctor to find out when you can safely work out again.

Exercising guarantees an energy boost. For the diehard exerciser, you need to know the difference between an energy boost with little fatigue from a good workout or utter exhaustion from needed rest and recovery. Grace to you. You've earned rest for a couple of days. This rest allows you to focus on expending extra energy toward adequate recovery so you won't get sick.

If you're the exerciser who may think this is crazy and it's a no brainer to rest, good. But you never know when you'll catch the exercise bug and need these grace reminders, too. Whether we're addicted to exercise or not, we all need grace.

Growing Roots
Day 235

Have you ever asked yourself the question, "Why do I do good things for my health and still see little results?" I have. But this last Sunday I had an "aha" moment. I've heard a lot of different sermons, but this one in particular stuck with me. The preacher was preaching on Jesus cursing the fig tree and how the disciples were thinking to themselves that it didn't work.

The disciples had been following Jesus and witnessing Him healing the sick and raising the dead, but when He cursed the fig tree nothing seemed to happen. What they didn't understand was, the fig tree had been cut off at the roots. The preacher gave the example of a fresh bouquet of flowers being so beautiful, but the truth is, they've been cut from their roots and will wither soon.

This sermon really spoke to me about fitness. We train day in and day out and don't really see what's truly going on inside. Little by little, we're establishing strong roots. Did you know that your muscle has memory? As you train, your muscle IS responding. I've had athletes that played a sport in high school or college get back into the game of fitness only to learn their bodies respond quicker than they thought they would. I've also witnessed people's discouragement and them quitting. What they don't realize is they are cutting their root source off and they will soon wither away.

Everything you're doing for your fitness is creating memory. It's working from the inside out, so doing what we know is good but can't see with our naked eye is working. Guaranteed, ALL ROOTS growing on the inside will bloom right before your very eyes. I challenge you to not cut yourself off at the roots.

Are You Anchored Down?
Day 236

Have you ever thought about how powerful an anchor is? Regardless of their size they all serve the same purpose, which is to keep a vessel from drifting. Without an anchor it is impossible to keep a boat where you want it, in particular when opposing forces such as wind and water come up against it. Commitment is the anchor for exercise. Without commitment we'll find ourselves adrift from including exercise in our lives.

I'm too tired. It's too late. It's too early. It's too hot. It's too cold. I don't have time. It's not doing any good so what's the point? These statements are some of the opposing forces we are met with daily when we are considering exercise. We've all said them, but when we're about to give in and not exercise for a day, we lose that commitment. Commitment is the strategy that anchors us to exercising one more day. The short commitment of time allotted daily will provide guaranteed long-term physical, mental, and emotional benefits.

I want to challenge you this week to anchor your exercise plans to commitment. As life brings its changes, it's easy to drift away from things that were once a priority. Keep exercise a priority. The short and long-term benefits from not drifting away will certainly be worth the commitment. Carry on my fitness friends; carry on!

A Healthy Foundation Produces Grace
Day 237

rest day

Have you ever heard someone say, "You're not getting any younger." The truth is, you really aren't getting any younger, and yet, it is possible to walk into your older years gracefully. It does take work, but it's worth your trouble. All this "good" work begins with your health and wellness foundation. You say you don't have a foundation? Everybody has one. The question is, "Is it a healthy foundation or an unhealthy foundation?"

A healthy foundation is defined as simply getting active, playing sports, and eating healthier. All three elements are essential, but today, I want to focus on the first. Getting active is so simple and so much more powerful than you know.

Becoming active can deeply affect you inside. You can make positive changes within your cells just by moving your body. Movement can change the way our DNA behaves. A single 20-minute workout appears to help tune up DNA, allowing muscles to work better and more efficiently. People who are genetically predisposed to obesity can trump their DNA by exercising for about 30 minutes, five days a week.

If your foundation is unhealthy, the good news is it can be improved IMMEDIATELY even if you've never exercised. Young, middle-aged, and mature individuals can all still benefit by beginning NOW. Sedentary people will actually fare better in percentage improvement gains relative to active people since they're starting from zero. Knowing this truth is all the more motivation to get moving.

I challenge you to become active TODAY and set yourself up to age gracefully. You never know what kind of benefits you'll produce by just taking a leap of faith. We're not getting any younger so let's tend to our foundation. It needs our constant care.

Dedicated or Obsessed?
Day 238

rest day

What is your first thought when I say the word dedicated? How about obsessed? Don't confuse dedication with obsession. Maintaining a fitness program requires dedication.

Dedication is a commitment to a plan that will produce a sustainable, healthy lifestyle. There is a fine line between being dedicated and being obsessed.

Obsession is where there is no peace in your fitness journey. You find yourself jumping from fad to fad, seeking out perfection, not ever happy with how you look or what you've already obtained. You set goals that are nearly impossible to achieve. If you do achieve an unrealistic goal, it's impossible to stay there. You may think you're getting somewhere, only to find that you're just chasing your tail.

Dedication will lead you down the path of freedom. You set goals that you can achieve, such as finding a sensible exercise regimen that is sustainable and can be peaceably maintained. You're setting yourself up to live a healthy lifestyle for the long run.

It's important to steer clear from frantic and fanatic behavior. Make sure you're on the track of exercising for a good cause: to be a better you. Being dedicated can keep you free from mental torment and maybe help your gym buddy that is obsessed.

I challenge you to discover the beautiful side of dedication. Guard yourself against becoming obsessed. Having the right mindset, you'll discover a freedom that will carry you through a lifetime.

Excess Salt, Anyone?
Day 239

Have you ever wondered about your salt intake? I'm a big observer of how many fats, proteins, or carbohydrates that are in a product, but not salt. Sure, I feel bloated or puffy after the consumption of salty foods but not too concerned, knowing a good sweat will get me back to normal.

I'd like to take a look together as to why we should be aware of consuming "too much salt."

You'll get thirsty a lot. Most people consuming too much sodium will find they're more thirsty than usual. The body needs extra fluids to help flush out the excess amount of sodium and restore its natural balance.

You'll start to swell up. Excess sodium interferes with the kidneys' ability to function. As a result, they cannot flush the fluid out of the body as efficiently as before. Some of the excess fluid gets squeezed into the spaces between cells where it cannot be discharged from the body, such as large bags under the eyes and swelling in the feet.

You may start to get headaches. The problem is dehydration can shrink the brain and cause it to shift away from the skull. This can induce pain until the brain swells back up to normal size once you drink enough fluids to rehydrate.

Do you need salt? Yes, the human body needs a certain amount of salt to function properly. The exact amount is up for debate since consumption varies in different areas of the world. The rule of thumb in the United States is under 2,300 milligrams per day. This is equal to about a half teaspoon.

I encourage you to be a constant learner because your body is ever changing. I challenge you not to grow weary, but instead be open to being all you can be.

The Facts ... Just the Facts
Day 240

 Today there's no fluff, encouragement, or motivational talk. I know it may not be easy to read, but I'm just giving you the facts.

Fact 1: In order to lose weight, you must burn off more calories than you consume. My advice is to be extremely active and enjoy food. Life is too short to be hungry.

Fact 2: In order to have a nice toned body, you must lift weights. The good news is there are many different ways to lift weights besides the traditional weightlifting in a gym. You can cut wood, do yard work, lift furniture, tackle do-it-yourself projects, or try home remodeling.

Fact 3: Exercise contributes to only 20% of what you need to maintain an optimal you, and yet it's definitely necessary for fitness.

Fact 4: Diet is 80% of the determining factor to reach the optimal you. Good nutrition really does show in weight, muscle tone, and even in the color of your skin.

Whenever I've fallen off the wagon, I simply begin again. I restart by doing the next right thing from the list above. Before I know it, I'm back on track until I fall again. I don't look at these fallen experiences like the end of the road, I simply remind myself to make a new start by using the facts.

I'll leave you with a guarantee. If you put forth any kind of effort to apply a fact from the list above, you'll get results. Sometimes we just need to face the facts. I encourage you to keep these facts handy for times when you feel overwhelmed or get off-track. You can make a fresh start when you apply the facts.

Yes, You Can
Day 241

Have you ever hit a lull in your fitness journey? I've hit many. I wish I could tell you that once you've made amazing strides forward in your journey, it's smooth sailing the rest of the way.

Quite the contrary; your health journey WILL have sharp, unexpected twists. Now is the time to decide to fasten your seatbelt and accept it. The problem is when an unexpected twist pops up, your mind begins to play tricks. The words, "I can't, I'm just so busy now, I'm bored, my body won't respond the way it used to," are LIES, LIES, LIES.

I'm here to tell you - yes you can. These types of thoughts can make you feel overwhelmed when you're trying to integrate healthy habits into your hectic schedule. If you find yourself in idle or off track, here are some healthy painless habits to try:

• Drink water throughout the day. This should be a daily reminder: water is an all-purpose wonder substance. It's great for your skin, your digestive system, and circulatory system. It also aids in weight loss and cellulite reduction.

• Exactly how much sugar are you consuming? Be aware of your current diet. I have a tendency to get off track and don't even realize it. Stay conscious of what you're putting in your mouth!

• Go to bed. If you're not getting the adequate amount of sleep you can gain weight. Your body heals and repairs itself as you sleep. If you're not getting your rest, your body will retain fluid and resist weight loss because it's fighting against itself to repair itself….GO TO BED.

Anything worthwhile takes effort. If you find yourself in a valley, I encourage you to begin to integrate one or all of these habits. Tell yourself…YES YOU CAN.

You Do You, Boo
Day 242

One of the best things about life is having the opportunity to be with family and friends. I'm sure we all have different family dynamics that bring out the best and worst in us. So, my "theme saying" lately is, "You Do You, Boo."

We all have different gifts and talents that reveal our individual personalities. When we come together with family and friends, we must adapt to all the personality differences that are involved. Instead of it being a dreaded experience, you can turn it around for good. The experience can actually be comical. Life is too short to get offended beyond repair.

I'm determined to shed all offense. I do know that's easier said than done. I choose to believe that no one means any harm. I like to handle anything anyone says with positivity and not give it another thought.

Same with fitness. When you're around a group of crossfitters, bootcampers, traditional training folks, barre die hards, kick boxers, boxers, Zumba lovers, yoga fanatics, walkers, runners, etc. … you need to just be who YOU are. Don't feel inadequate being a bootcamp person when your bestie is a crossfitter. You must simply soar in your own niche and just "do you, Boo."

Life is a lot more peaceful when we allow everyone to be who they are. I'm here to tell you, "You do you, Boo." The fitness arena is too big for anyone not to find anything they personally enjoy. Give yourself a lot of grace, as you revel in your perfect niche. Make sure to give those around you the same freedom in return. We want everyone to love exercise and flourish in what works for each of us.

S.M.A.R.T.
Day 243

I'm in the middle of a goal, so I've been thinking about it a lot lately. I'm not eating cakes, pies, cookies, ice cream, chocolate, or candy. I first set out to do it for a month, but I undeniably feel amazingly better so I extended it another month. It would be logical to quit sweets forever.

You must be smart about how you set goals. If you make your fitness journey a lifestyle, you'll experience victories and defeats. You mustn't park your tent in either place. Saying you'll never do something again means more than likely you'll do it again.

This acronym, S.M.A.R.T., has helped me:

SPECIFIC: Set up guardrails by defining clear parameters for your goal. For example: My goal is no cakes, pies, cookies, ice cream, chocolate, or candy. These guardrails won't allow me to justify an all natural cookie for a cookie.

MEASURABLE: Let's assume your goal is to lose 10 pounds; it's week three and you've only lost 3 1/2 pounds. Make sure you celebrate the small victory of 3 1/2 pounds.

ATTAINABLE: Make sure your goal is reasonable and can be reached. Being reasonable in attaining your particular goal involves all three of the above, together.

REALISTIC: There's no better way to fail than to set your goal too high. Keep it realistic. Setting out to lose 60 pounds in a month is NOT a realistic number. You'll be discouraged and extremely frustrated.

TIMELY: There must be a clear start and end date. I challenge you to set an ending so you won't be left always wanting. This journey is an endless one. To stay encouraged, set a beginning and end.

Overtraining DOES Exist
Day 244

rest day Strangely enough, overtraining DOES exist and it will compromise results. I was just talking to someone who said they've been an avid endurance biker for years, but that it has now put his heart into AFib. His doctor told him that biking like he has (maximum intensity for hours) places the same stress on your heart as if you were a couch potato overdoing it on their first workout.

How can you tell if you're overtraining? Your body will give you signs.

Here are some symptoms:

For the regular gym attender, you may feel shockingly reluctant to head to the gym, and if you do get there, lifting (for example) seems much more difficult. You will be unable to match your usual weights, sets, or reps.

Muscle soreness is common, and by that I don't mean the usual delayed onset muscle soreness (DOMS) that invariably follows a good gym session (usually in a day or two). In overtraining, one feels heavy and just sort of achy all over.

You experience chronic fatigue. The person who has chronic fatigue takes far longer to recover from an exercise bout. The simple task of walking could set back your energy level for days.

How do you treat overtraining? The first thing is lots of rest. If you're genuinely over-trained, don't go back into the gym (or run, or whatever other intense exercise training you do) until you feel completely well.

Nutrition can play a large role in recovery from overtraining. Increasing your protein intake, such as a larger helping of lean meat or fish, at least once on most days each week, will assist in the recovery process.

I challenge you to listen to your body and get exactly what is needed to thrive at your best potential.

Proud to Present Client #3's Testimony
Day 245

rest day

Here's her journey: "Started taking classes with Jade in August. My 'before' picture is actually the day after the first class I ever took. My 'after' picture is from April. I used to just go on Thursdays to work out, but a few years ago I started going Mondays as well. My highest weight was right at 200 lbs. Currently I'm around 160 lbs. I did my first 5k in June.

So far this year, I have completed two 5k's and I'm signed up for three more. I go to the YMCA. I'm getting ready to start kickboxing. I don't really have a set diet. I have been trying to watch my portion sizes and stay away from sweets. I don't eat chocolate due to lactose intolerance. I think being more active has helped a lot in maintaining my weight loss so far. My goal weight is around 130 lbs."

Client #3's success began with one class. Then by adding a little more activity and setting some small realistic diet goals along the way (portion control and making better food choices), BAM … Seven years later, she's on FIRE, looking FABULOUS, and has hit her desired weight of 130 lbs.

The exciting part about it all is that fitness is a big part of her life. As her trainer, I've watched her grow and develop in many different ways. She's like a beautiful butterfly changed forever. There's a lot to be said for not being in such a hurry all of the time.

You've got your own fitness success to be had. I challenge you to keep at your goals. See you on video! I'm excited to help you.

Weekend Eating
Day 246

I don't know about you, but when Friday rolls around, I'm ready to chow down. That's OK to a certain extent, but to do it to the point of no return can destroy everything we've worked so hard to accomplish during our workweek.

The structure of the workweek can be extremely conducive to maintaining good eating habits. The workweek provides a very predictable daily routine; it's easier to plan meals and snacks. But when the weekend comes, all that structure disappears and leads many people to make unhealthy eating choices.

Examples:

It's party time. Alcohol lowers your inhibitions, making it more likely that you'll make poor food choices. Or you might eat when you're not really hungry. If you're going to drink, you might consider wine. A glass of red wine has health benefits.

I've been good all week - I deserve a treat! Following a healthy eating plan is not about never eating high calorie foods you enjoy. Instead of depriving yourself of your favorites all week long only to overdo it on the weekend, plan a few small treats throughout the week.

TV or movie time. There's absolutely nothing wrong with wanting to take a break and enjoy a movie at home or the theater. Just be smart about how you handle the snacking portion of your relaxation time.

I'll bet you could come up with a list of your own. I challenge you to continue setting small, achievable goals. Constantly work toward them. I encourage you to do what you can. If you're making progress, you're winning. Small steps really do pay off in the long run. Don't let go of the rope; hang on during the weekend. You can do it.

Frustrated
Day 247

I had a client share her struggle of eating all the right things for the past 20 days without losing a pound. As she shared, others in the class spoke up and said she looks like she has lost weight. It's not just about weight loss. We must embrace that if we're putting forth effort, things are guaranteed to change.

My precious client, for instance, didn't lose a pound, BUT she looked a lot leaner. Her focus was on the scale, but as soon as a fitness friend asked her if her clothes are fitting different, she said, "YES." Her wrong focus left her frustrated to the point of tears.

Her struggle got me thinking about the term, "fat thermostat." A fat thermostat is your brain's set point to function similarly, maintaining a consistent weight and fat level through interactions of hormones. Each body has a weight it fights to maintain. When an individual wants to change their weight, the body requires time to come to terms with changing the internal fat thermostat.

I always tell my clients that have gained or even lost weight quickly that your own body will fight you to get back to the particular weight your body is used to maintaining.

The good news is the fat thermostat can be changed by an individual doing something that causes the brain to change its settings (like eating clean and exercising) for weight control. This is accomplished over time. If you don't give up and hang in there to give your body time to internally change its fat thermostat, once it has, you'll start seeing progress on a weekly, if not daily, basis.

I encourage you to continue exercising and eating right, and don't be fooled … placing your frustrations at bay, you're producing results, guaranteed …

What Happens When I Exercise?
Day 248

I'd like to take a very technical topic and bring it to you in simple terms. What specifically happens to your body when you exercise? The biological effects that occur are fascinating. Your body is affected from head to toe when you exercise.

Muscles: As soon as you begin any type of vigorous movement, your muscles will require the use of sugar and adenosine triphosphate (also known as ATP) for contraction and movement. As soon as your body gets a clue that you're not stopping any time soon, it will create more ATP. ATP is like fuel, and in order for you to produce more ATP, your body needs extra oxygen.

Your breathing increases to supply more oxygen, and your heart starts pumping more blood to your muscles. During intense exercise, a metabolic byproduct is produced. This byproduct is called lactic acid. Lactic acid causes muscle fatigue and post-exercise muscle soreness caused from tiny muscle tears.

These tiny muscle tears are actually what make your muscles grow bigger and stronger as they heal. This is the very reason recovery time is essential! With proper rest and hydration, you'll be even stronger for your next workout.

Interestingly, exercising regularly will promote the growth of new brain cells, too. A number of neurotransmitters are also triggered, such as endorphins and serotonin. These particular neurotransmitters are well-known for their role in mood control. Exercise is one of the most effective prevention and treatment strategies for depression.

Now that you know what happens when you exercise, you'll embrace all the wonderful side effects. Being a little out of breath makes for stronger lungs and heart. Being a little sore develops pretty muscles. We are given one body in a lifetime. Believe you're worth it. Keep it in motion.

The Three P's of Fitness
Day 249

 Let's categorize our health and wellness into three "P" words. These three words must be considered. If we don't digest all three of these "P" words, we can't really keep health a priority.

The first "P" is Personal. Take "The Biggest Loser," a T.V. show from years ago. The participants losing weight always got emotional at some point. When people decide to do something to better themselves, many things surface from a person's past, such as disappointments, defeats, trauma, childhood wounds, etc. For these reasons, we need to buckle up with understanding and press forward with an overcoming drive.

The second "P" is Precise. I had a friend way back in my 20's that was a precision welder. I would visit him at his shop and stand in awe of how he worked on massively huge pieces of equipment to precisely mold a tiny segment. We're like the tiny segments in this big massive world. We're special and unique individuals in constant need of precise tuning.

The last "P" is Purpose. We're born for such a time as this. We all have a specific, special purpose on this earth to fulfill. If we don't have our health and wellness in check or a priority, we're unable to carry out our God-given purpose to our best ability. If we don't feel good, how are we to give our best? Fitness enables purpose.

Think about your own "P's" of fitness. Reflect on your personal lives and ask yourselves what might be holding you back. What precision tuning does your fitness need to become an even better version of yourself?

Reflect on what you're doing and ask yourself if you're doing it with excellence.

My Testimony
Day 250

When I say my passion is fitness, I mean it has truly been my lifelong "friend" that has helped me cope with all the ups and downs of my life. Ever since I can remember, one of my most prominent characteristics has been my physical strength. I was never a good student due to learning disabilities, but I could arm wrestle the football team and throw the cheerleaders up in the air (just like the guys do now but this was before there were guys on a squad). We all gravitate toward our strengths in order to be accepted by others, so I buried myself in exercise to cover my learning challenges.

At thirty years old I was at a crossroads. My dad was a great help through this period. He offered me to live with him short term while I attended Massage Therapy School, with a couple of rules. His biggest rule was I had to go to church with him every Sunday.

My first church attendance, my sister and I had gone out the night before, so I was still in party mode, and I had no idea what was about to happen that Sunday morning. I answered the altar call, bowed my head, and said a prayer with a quaint group of people. Still half lit from the night before, I opened my eyes and did a 180 turn with my life right then and there. This was my "Right Side Up" moment. Ever since that day back in 1997, I have never been the same.

You may be wondering why I write about my story of fitness and faith and how it relates to you. None of us are exempt from hard times, so I challenge you to think about what has gotten you through.

Physical Activity vs Exercise
Day 251

A client shared that she's walking an additional six miles each day and not losing any weight. Due to her being in incredible shape, I immediately knew that her extra walking is not considered "exercise time" but instead is considered "physical activity." There is a difference between exercise time and physical activity. You'll hear me refer to "physical activity" as "active rest."

Exercise time is a planned, structured, repetitive, and intentional movement intended to improve or maintain physical fitness. In order for it to be considered "exercise time," your planned, structured time must consist of frequency (3-5 days per week), intensity (60-85% of maximum heart rate), and time (20-60 minutes of continuous rhythmic activities).

Physical activity ("active rest") is movement that is carried out by the skeletal muscles that requires energy but not with great intensity. Any movement you do is considered physical activity. Depending on your fitness level, your "exercise time" and your "physical activity" will vary.

For instance, for my very fit client who is walking an extra 6 miles, walking is considered physical activity. For a sedentary client, who's just starting a new exercise program, walking 6 miles is considered "exercise time."

We need both exercise time and physical activity time to become the best we can be. Adding physical activity positively contributes to overall health and well-being. Be encouraged that all activity is great for you.

Your bodies are made to move. I challenge you to not take your body for granted; it is a God-given GIFT. If you're extremely fit, applaud yourself. If you're sedentary, no worries! You can simply begin by finding something to do to be physically active and work up to a structured exercise time. All movement helps more than you know, even if the scale isn't moving. You are reaping benefits.

The Thrill of Expectancy – the Agony of Defeat
Day 252

What were your expectations when you started exercising? Expectations say, "if I do this then I should get that." The box we place our expectations in keeps us in just that...A Box. Our box of expectations may look like this: "That's all I want," "I need to reach this before a certain date," "It has to come off," "If I don't reach my goal I'm gonna quit," or "My exercise will give me the confidence to do this or do that." Do any of those sayings sound familiar? The very specific thing we are aiming for can sometimes get in the way of seeing the results that are surfacing.

Ways on how to keep the thrill and squash agony:

1. Lay aside perceived expectations. If you're 6'4", long, lean, and made for the basketball court, don't set your sails on developing Arnold Schwarzenegger biceps.

2. For all of us ladies, if the good Lord blessed you with CrossFit legs, don't set your heart on size 2 pants. Let's be open to receiving results that transpire no matter what size we are.

3. We all want to look like we did at the age we felt and looked our best. That longing can take you down a road of agony. How about being the best you can be at whatever age you are right now?

So remember, stay open to the window of continual opportunity. Open yourself up to the greater picture. Don't begin your fitness adventure in a box. True lifelong health and wellness can only be found outside of the box. Now, go forward fully in the thrill of expectancy, not allowing any agony of any unmet and unrealistic expectation to get you off track.

Welcome the Distraction
Day 253

Ever since I can remember, I've been weight conscious. I've carried the childhood lies of being "Fat, White, and Ugly" that only led to lots of wasted, unwanted, and self-destructive years. So, needless to say, I've tried every diet in the book, but really to no avail.

My family has always been characteristically thin. I'm considered a normal build, but always felt big in comparison to my family. One diet, I tried to follow my little sister around and eat like she did for the day. I thought since she was thin, she wouldn't eat a lot. Well, I was right; she barely ate. I was starving and kept asking her, "Aren't you hungry?" That diet didn't last.

Another diet suggestion my skinny sister tried sharing was what she calls "welcome the distraction." When her kids were little, their needs pulled her away from the dinner table. She learned by the time she returned to the table she wasn't hungry anymore. Yep, I tried that, too. I learned that welcoming the distraction only made me determined to finish. I'd welcome the distraction alright, but found myself gravitating right back to the kitchen to finish what I started, despite any distraction.

My new big thing that has brought me some victory is being aware of my thoughts. It takes serious happenstance for us to stop using food as a tool for comfort. I don't use food for fuel consciously. I'm one of those who uses food as comfort. But by golly, I'm getting better and I'm determined to never quit.

I encourage you to keep on seeking and never stop. Interview people that use food for fuel and learn from them. Welcome the distraction. Who knows? It may work for you.

What if You Didn't?
Day 254

 We're quick to the punch when it comes to putting off exercise. We have a hundred excuses why we don't. When the day gets hectic, exercise usually takes a back seat real quickly. In general, exercise has a negative connotation. Let's use some reverse psychology. What if we didn't exercise? It's risky business…if we don't.

Here are some truths we may inevitably face if we don't exercise:

Inactivity is usually followed by weight and blood pressure problems. When you don't move, either by choice or due to injury, you burn fewer calories each day. Some of the primary benefits of exercise include maintaining a healthy weight and regulating blood pressure.

Loss of bone strength occurs due to inactivity. Sitting or laying around all day makes you weak. Unless you continuously use the major muscle groups in your body, they do not strengthen. Bones also lose density. The lack of weight-bearing exercise plays a role in osteoporosis or brittle bones. Your body responds to the demands you put on it, so if you don't exercise, your muscles and bones weaken with time.

Inactivity usually accompanies weak mental health. Lack of exercise can lead to a lessened sense of well-being. Your body loses muscle tone and strength, resulting in low self-esteem. Low self-esteem could lead to social isolation and bad eating habits. Vigorous aerobic exercise such as swimming or running stimulates your body to release endorphins, which reduce depression.

What if you DID exercise? Type 2 diabetes could be obsolete. Knee pain could be eliminated. Back pain could come to an end. Little to no energy could be reversed to Speedy Gonzales energy. Weak muscles could be converted to Popeye the Sailor Man strength. Don't be fooled - exercise affects our health in big ways.

Major Calorie Burners
Day 255

In one of my classes, we discussed the muscles of the body. I tell all of my clients, "Training legs is training your major calorie burners."

When I began to have hip trouble about five years ago, I thought, "OH NO!" What am I going to do if I can't train my major calorie burners? Our recent class discussion on muscles challenged me regarding the largest muscle in the body, being the *gluteus maximus* and not the quadriceps, because the quadriceps is a group of four smaller muscles that make up the "quadriceps group."

I had to question myself. It only makes sense for the largest muscle to burn the most calories. Right? The larger the muscle, the more energy it requires, so we mustn't ignore the largest muscle in the body – your *gluteus maximus*. Going forward, I can't omit the *gluteus maximus*.

I learned in order to burn the maximum amount of calories, we actually need to do exercises that simultaneously recruit both upper leg muscles and glute muscles, done intensely.

Here are some exercises that achieve that goal:

Squats with a free barbell: The Squat is a full body compound exercise.

Deadlift: The deadlift will strengthen every bone in your body, challenge every muscle across your posterior chain (all the muscles that run from your neck to your heels), and test your grip strength and core stability to the absolute max.

Leg press: This particular exercise is performed by lying on the floor with feet on the straight bar.

Lunges: Always engage your core. Step forward with one leg, lowering your hips until both knees are bent at about a 90-degree angle.

Challenge yourself. Burn the maximum amount of calories. Remember, you must engage the gluteus muscle group, quad group, and hamstring group simultaneously with intense exertion.

Keep Your Eyes on the Prize
Day 256

We must constantly keep our eyes on the prize, count our blessings, look at the glass half full, and stay encouraged about our own personal health.

We've all been discouraged about our health and wellness at one time or another. We all long to be successful in this journey. Over the years, in helping others and in my own fitness journey, I've discovered it's all about the small steps. Lasting fitness success comes about via one small change at a time.

Having a positive mindset is first in making small changes to improve your health. You'll find yourself encouraged and desiring to do more. You can master a small habit to where it becomes second nature. I've done this with drinking water. The habit of drinking water has kept my body hydrated for better results. One habit becomes routine, then another good habit can be implemented (walking daily). As you continue to add one habit to another good habit this will steadily move you toward big change.

Changing old behaviors takes work, so you need a good reason to make a new habit worth your effort. Then you must support your new habit. Tell a trusted friend or family member what you're doing, and ask them to remind you why you're in this game.

Pursuing better health takes time. The small-habit approach won't work overnight. But it can keep you on track without the jarring impact of a huge life change. Adding one small habit after another leads you to powerful, healthy habits you can use to keep your health in check.

Each time you follow through with a small habit, you build confidence. You feel more in control. A lifestyle change develops almost unaware. I encourage you to be victory-minded. Victory is earned one step at a time.

Is There a Formula?
Day 257

Is there a formula for the perfect body? If there was, we'd all use that formula and walk around sharing it with all who are in need of help. Even though there isn't a formula to having "the perfect body," there are guidelines.

Again, these guidelines are cardiovascular, resistance, and flexibility training. I encourage you to study all three areas and find your specific formula.

Although the above guidelines are the keys in finding your personal formula, it's through trial and error. Each individual needs to discover what works for them and what doesn't. If you've tried all of the above and nothing seems to work, simply continue moving forward doing the next right thing and you will reap success, guaranteed.

The biggest hurtle to overcome is accepting your fitness journey has no destination. You must accept your health and wellness is an ongoing journey, just like eating your next meal. I encourage you to embrace every new day with the excitement of learning something new and fun about yourself and fitness.

As your personal trainer, I'm here to help you find your perfect formula. I'm just a text away.

Walking Your Way Out of Depression
Day 258

rest day I received a testimony from a client of mine about how she walked her way out of depression. Gyms closed for a long time during the pandemic, and she had to find another way to keep herself fit. She found a walking app on her phone, tried it, and found that she really enjoyed it. In so doing, she says she "walked her way out of depression."

For good reason, I'd like to share some benefits of walking.

Walking will improve your mood. Walking can decrease levels of anger and hostility, and it can promote feelings of well-being, especially when you're going for a stroll through some greenery or soaking in a bit of sunlight.

Walking will improve your digestion and help you burn calories and lose weight. Regular walking can help improve your body's response to insulin, which can help reduce belly fat. Daily walking increases metabolism by burning extra calories and preventing muscle loss, which is particularly important as we get older.

It can even help alleviate joint pain. Contrary to what you might think, pounding the pavement can actually help improve your range of motion and mobility. That's because walking increases blood flow to tense areas and helps strengthen the muscles surrounding the joints.

Walking can help you live longer. Adults between the ages of 70 and 90 who often left their houses and were physically active lived longer than those who didn't. Staying active and connected to loved ones can also provide emotional support.

The benefits of walking are endless and worth every single step. Walking your way out of depression can put a dance in your step. Who knew you could walk your way to a happier and healthier you? I challenge you to try it and find out for yourself.

Variety is the Spice of Life
Day 259

rest day As you carry out your fitness regimen, making it a priority, you'll discover over time that your workouts need something. Sometimes, you might not be sure what that "something" could be. Our bodies are amazing machines. They figure out what new demand we place on them and then adapt to the physical tasks we put them through really quickly.

One benefit is that normal tasks becomes easier, along with your workouts. When this is occurring, it's time to implement change. Muscle confusion is a great something to add to your routine for change. Muscle confusion is implementing new exercises into your existing routines to keep your muscles guessing and your body responding nicely to the new work required.

There are several ways to keep your body on the cutting edge. During resistance training, a pyramid workout is one technique that starts off light the first set, heavier the second, then tops out heaviest during the third set, ending by working your way back to light weight. Calisthenics can be implemented in between sets of dumbbell work to keep the body awake.

Another way (depending on physical ability) is to incorporate explosive movements that are safe and controlled throughout your resistance training workout. Explosive movements are quick reps that fatigue the muscle.

As you accept the fact that variety is one factor to meeting your next fitness level, you can look forward to trying new things and figuring out what works best for your particular body. You then feel revived and can get excited about renewing first found love of exercise again. If you've never experienced that love for exercise, it's not too late to find it.

I encourage you to find variety so you can keep your body jumping, responsive, and strong.

Are You Staying Hopeful?
Day 260

Staying hopeful on your fitness journey is crucial. The saying, "Life is 10 percent what happens to you and 90 percent how you respond to it" by Lou Holtz is so true. To transform your thinking is to transform your life. This is done through POSITIVE THINKING.

You'll read this over and over again. It can't be said enough. Positive thinking along your fitness journey is a must for reaching what you long to achieve. How you think of your fitness literally transforms you. For instance, if you think positively about the benefits of healthy foods, new fitness classes, or exercise, you'll be more likely to stay on the right path with patience and endurance.

Sure, you can rest or eat a cheat meal, but the bulk of your thinking should be focused on the awesome things your fitness journey has to offer. There are so many negative things you can attach yourself to in this world. Advertisers know if you're constantly being told that Coke will satisfy your thirst, the next time you go into a store and see a bottle of Coke, it'll be the first thing you'll pick up.

The same is true for advertisements of body image. Throughout your day, you see models on billboards, in magazines, or on social media, and then turn on the T.V. in the evening only to find more self expectations. This leaves you with subliminal messages of negativity and insecurity.

How can you stay positive with these subconscious messages? You must be intentional about thinking optimistic thoughts and creating your own hopeful mindsets. This is done by repetition and requires hard work. It's no easy task. Anything worthwhile takes hard work and determination to achieve. Staying on this journey isn't for the faint of heart.

Endorphin Junkie
Day 261

We need to eat to survive and thrive. Food is our fuel source and a necessity to sustain life. But have you ever looked at the meal you're about to eat and asked yourself the question, "What's all the hype?" I've often wondered why food is such a big deal. Why do people, such as myself, want to stuff themselves beyond the point of full?

There are many reasons an individual eats food beyond its design for fuel. One reason is our brains release extra endorphins that literally alter our brain chemistry. The extra endorphin release results in a euphoric feeling. This feeling becomes a fix as we turn to food like a trusted friend.

Some of us eat for an endorphin rush and not always for fuel. Sugar is the number one go-to for an endorphin rush. The problem is thirty minutes later you crash, becoming lethargically nonproductive.

Another go-to for an endorphin rush is complex carbohydrates. These include rice, potatoes, pastas, and breads. It's hard to find a decent meal without hitting carbohydrate overload. A telltale sign you've tapped into a rush is thirty minutes later you're ready for a nap. Most people have experienced this on Thanksgiving Day.

A great alternative to releasing endorphins is exercise. It's a fix that won't leave you feeling down with extra weight to lose. Exercise releases serotonin, which is considered a natural pain reliever (aka endorphins). A simple exercise class is guaranteed to release this natural opiate that relieves pain and can also relieve stress or enhance life's experiences guilt free.

Let's say bye bye to food endorphin fixes that leave us in a mound of guilt. Let's eat food the way it was designed, for fuel. I challenge you to be a healthy endorphin junkie.

Being Organized Can Lead to Weight Loss
Day 262

Yes, being organized can actually lead to weight loss. Sometimes I'm a bit too organized. I lack excitement in my current season of life. Looking back despite the season, being organized has helped me tremendously in staying on track.

I encourage you to organize your time. You're probably more organized than you realize. You have to be on time to work and leave on time. Your kids have to be picked up from school on time. They have sports practice, appointments, etc. at specific times on specific days.

Maybe you don't have kids. Whatever you're into, you know what day and time to be at your next event. We know that we have organizational skills. Let's take the same approach to our schedule for weight loss.

Scheduling your workouts: pick a specific time each week to review your calendar for the days ahead, and schedule your workouts accordingly. Don't forget to factor in travel time to and from a gym.

Planning your work week meals: figure out where and when you'll be eating meals, what foods you'll need to have on hand, and when you'll have time to cook. Be proactive, not reactive.

Good bed time habits: go to bed. Sleep deprivation interferes with weight loss by messing with hormones and hanging on to unwanted fluid and weight. Good sleep is when your body repairs itself and builds muscle.

I challenge you to be organized. The Bible even says so. In Habakkuk 2:2-3 it says, "Write the vision and make it plain on tablets, that he may run who reads it. For the vision is yet for the appointed time, but at the end it will speak, and it will not lie. Though it tarries, wait for it: because it will surely come, it will not tarry."

Lose Five Pounds Quick!
Day 263

I know losing weight can be a complex matter, but there's a really easy way to drop five pounds. The answer…eliminating the calories you drink. If you're a juice/soda drinker, you can lose up to five pounds if you eliminate the calories in what you drink.

When my daughter was a teenager and went to her prom, she decided to eat healthy leading up to her big evening. She wanted me to buy her some cranberry juice, thinking it's a healthy move. Sure, fruit juices have some benefits, but there are other ways to reap those benefits without the high calories.

Eating fruit is a much healthier choice than drinking it. This is because it takes a whole lot more fruit to produce a cup of juice, which therein lies the extra calories. For example, 3 cups of raw cranberries makes up 1 cup of cranberry juice. That's a lot of cranberries to eat.

Same is true with other fruit juices. There are anywhere between three and six apples, depending on the size and type of apples, to equal one cup (8 oz.) of apple juice. Orange juice is a popular way to start the day. It can take up to four medium oranges to produce one cup of orange juice. That's a lot of oranges to eat before you start the day.

Two cans of soda per day adds approximately 24 to 35 pounds of fat per year, depending on body size, age, habits, etc. Some people (weighing in at 140 pounds) have reported that by giving up two cans of soda per day, without exercise, they lost 20 pounds in six months. Now, that's good news.

The bottom line is to not drink your calories. I challenge you to eat your calories, don't drink them.

Are You Walking Properly?
Day 264

When my family heads out for the day, my girls run to the shoe closet and throw on the nearest pair of shoes they can find and they're out the door. I, on the other hand, have to figure out where we are going and what we're doing so I can put on the appropriate footwear.

It's one thing to wear proper shoes, but did you know there's a proper way to walk?

To evaluate your walk, try moving your ankles through their complete range of motion. From a standing position, step forward landing squarely on the heel of your foot. Next, roll forward onto the ball of the foot, and raise the heel and push off with your big toe.

To see how this heel-to-toe motion should feel, try sitting on a chair with your legs extended straight out in front of you with your toes pointing straight up to the ceiling. With your left foot, bring your toes back toward you so your heel is extended and your foot is flexed. With your right foot, push your toes forward as if pushing on the air with the ball of your foot and big toe. Reverse the positions of your feet, moving back and forth for one minute.

This is the ideal motion for walking, but most of us don't walk perfectly, Therefore, you will more than likely notice some burning or tension in your shins or calves when you do it. This sensation means that the muscles where you feel the soreness are underused, and you may need to do some strengthening and stretching exercises.

Walking is good exercise when done correctly. So, the next time you get up, I challenge you to evaluate your walk to see if there is any room for improvement.

Too Much of This Won't Take Care of That
Day 265

rest day Is eating too much of a good thing not good for us? To answer that question, it's important to understand how the body functions during exercise. It is good to know what exactly your body needs whether you have or have not been exercising for a while.

During exercise, your body is in a performance state. If you aren't exercising, you're like a parked car ready for performance at any time. Also like a car, your body requires different fuel based on your high, medium, or low performance level. Therefore, what you eat becomes an important factor in meeting the daily performance demand your body requires.

If you under eat, you aren't going to function very well either. The same goes if you overeat. Like with a car, placing the right amount of fluids in the right places is essential. You can't put antifreeze, oil, windshield wiper fluid, or brake fluid in a car's gas tank and expect it to run properly. The same goes with bad gas; the car just won't work properly.

Even if you can determine good food from bad food, you still need to experiment to find the food that agrees best with your own body. For example, eating onions of any kind makes me feel sick to my stomach. So although onions are good for me, my body doesn't perform well eating them.

I challenge you to vary your food intake levels and the types of foods you eat and see how they affect your diet and exercise. You can try new ways or repeat old ways to find what works best for your particular performance level. When you find your own unique mix, it will be a discovery that lasts a lifetime.

Help! Where is this Extra Weight Coming From?
Day 266

Where is this extra weight coming from? This is a perplexing question to answer because we all differ in so many ways. Two out of three Americans are now either overweight or obese. Contrary to popular belief, obesity is not always the result of eating too many calories and not exercising enough. There are some other environmental and lifestyle factors that may play a role in not losing weight, or give some answers where the extra weight may be coming from.

Meat. Meat companies add growth hormones to fatten up their livestock. These growth enhancing drugs have been proven to affect an individual's health.

Artificial sweeteners. The business of artificial sweeteners is built on the idea that no or low-calorie sugar substitutes will help you lose weight. Unfortunately, this simply isn't true. Artificially sweetened "diet" foods and beverages tend to stimulate your appetite, increase cravings for carbs, and stimulate fat storage and weight gain.

Junk food marketing and falling prey to the wrong types of foods. Advertisement even deceives people to convince them a food is good for you, but in reality it's not. This issue of junk food marketing is particularly detrimental when aimed at kids. Kids are literally being deceived and manipulated into destroying their health by junk food companies seeking revenue.

As you can see, other factors contribute to weight problems. Simply eating fewer calories and exercising may not work very well because not all calories are the same. Instead of focusing on calories, let's address the "quality of the foods" we eat.

Create a list of healthy options. I challenge you to be cautious of advertisement. Keep in mind that whole, unadulterated "real foods" are rarely if ever advertised. Stay alert and on guard of what may be the real culprit to a weight gain.

The Unique You
Day 267

You are unique. Read that again. You are unique. Most people don't believe that and become their own worst enemies. If you are reading this and are happy with your uniqueness, consider yourself blessed.

Ever since I can remember, I've always battled demons who convinced me that I was fat, white, and ugly. These three simple words have kept me bound most of my life. They make me see everyone, from 8 to 88, as prettier, thinner, and tanner than me. I know this sounds vain and senseless, but I'll bet your lies would sound senseless, too, if you shared them.

Let's speak truth. I don't want to be prettier, thinner, and tanner. I simply want to live free. My broken record began playing in my mind during puberty, got really loud in my twenties, and got too loud in my thirties. Unable to fight any longer, I found myself in a counseling chair. Now in my mid-fifties, when that broken record wants to start, I have the ability to turn it off. I want to help you get control of your lies and broken records, too.

Movement is a great way to counteract lies in that it builds up determination. It helps us focus on accepting ourselves so we can get on with life. In accepting ourselves, we can learn to accept and love others the way God intended.

We have a unique physique waiting to be discovered. So regardless of how we see ourselves, we must push through the lies that hold us back and just move.

I challenge you to connect with others. Share a walk. Discover the uniqueness in others. Yes, something that simple can begin to manifest the unique you. So disregard the lies you listen to and celebrate the uniqueness in you.

What Does Health & Wellness Freedom Look Like?
Day 268

I've been wanting to write about what freedom looks like on a health and wellness journey, but I could never really place my finger on exactly what to write. Usually, when I have a topic, I have a general idea, but this time was different.

I kept thinking about how to begin, then it came to me. … I don't have the words because I don't have freedom mastered. I still struggle a lot. I've spent my whole life's journey trying to attain freedom with my eating and exercise. All my life I've excelled in athletics but had deep-seated issues with either too much or too little food. After my high school and college days of cheerleading, fitness competitions, track, tennis, and cross country running ended, I became obsessed with my exercise routine.

My issues led me to a fair share of counseling throughout my life. One particular counselor diagnosed me with exercise bulimia. I would eat excessively then exercise just as excessively. Previously, I would starve myself all day long then get up at 2 a.m. to eat that one golden meal I saved. This eating was always followed by running excessively the next day.

I had to get my run, weight training, or some form of exercise in before I could enjoy my own children, family, or friends. My solution to my exercise obsession was to get up early enough to work out before my husband and kids got up. I was filled with obsession, fear, and guilt. I was consumed with disappointment about the way I looked.

What does freedom in health and wellness look like? To me, it means to never quit or stop learning, because being challenged in life is inevitable; being defeated is optional.

Proper Positions
Day 269

Standing is something you do without thinking, like breathing. There's a proper way to breathe. There's also a proper way to stand. When you first learned to stand as a toddler, it was through trial and error. With practice, you learned to balance over your feet and then learned how to propel yourself forward with steps. After some spills and awkward moments, standing and walking eventually became habitual.

Most people subconsciously developed poor habits and never modified that learned technique. For example, my daughter walked on her tippy toes most of the time as a toddler. Even today, as a young adult, she battles to keep her heels on the floor.

Today, I'd like to share how to stand aligned and balanced.

Standing Correctly. A proper standing position is first to balance your body over your feet. Your spine should be aligned over your pelvis, with your weight evenly distributed between your feet. Many people stand with more weight over one foot or with their weight over only part of their feet.

While standing, become aware of your feet. You should feel even pressure on the balls of your big toes, little toes, and heels. This is the tripod of your foot. If you feel more pressure on one of these points, you are not in alignment.

Proper Foot Position. When standing, your feet should be parallel and at least 3 inches apart. Because the angle of the ankle joint varies among people, a slight turnout of the ankle (no more than 10 degrees) may be present.

One last fact – standing is good, but standing for an extended period of time can hinder blood flow. The human body was designed for constant movement. I encourage you to take frequent, brief, walking breaks during your day when possible.

Fourth Quarter

Daily Inspirations for Fitness

I See the Finish Line

Days 270 - 366

**Scan the QR Code for each day
to take you to a companion
YouTube Video Workout**

Fitness 101
Day 270

The simple building blocks of fitness success are easy to forget in lieu of the latest and greatest fitness craze. These tips might seem simplistic and elementary, but they're important for any trainee to revisit and utilize.

Here are some Fitness 101 reminders:

1. Have fun. You're more apt to stay consistent; if you're not having fun with your fitness, it's easy to lose interest.

2. Set goals. Maybe you want to fit into a smaller dress size, decrease your body fat percentage, cut your mile time, or set a new lifting PR. That goal will help you stay focused and on the path to success.

3. Drink water. While the reminder to drink water may sound unnecessary and obvious, many people often mistake their thirst for hunger.

4. Protein. While exact daily protein requirements vary by individual and goal, you need enough to maintain and build lean muscle mass. A diet that's rich in protein will help you feel fuller for longer while refueling your muscles post-workout.

5. Vegetables. The more colors you eat the better. Enjoy the variety.

6. Food prep. When it comes to meals, don't be caught off guard. The more you can plan ahead, the better. I always have a healthy snack with me so I won't be tempted to pull into a fast food place.

7. Mix it up. Many dedicated gym-goers fall into a workout rut. Make some changes for new challenges.

My momma always taught me to "keep it simple sweetheart (K.I.S.S.)," with fashion that is. I've found the same thing true when it comes to fitness. Keep it simple sweetheart, because we've got some exercising to do for a lifetime!!

Working Through Sadness
Day 271

Not long ago, I lost my dog of nine years. I experienced a true facet of sadness. I know she was just a dog, but it gave me some understanding of what it would be like to lose a loving mate or child. I'm not belittling the grief of a human soul to a furry friend. I could only imagine the pain of losing a loved one.

The hardest part is missing her unconditional love. She was harmless. She was always happy to see me, go anywhere, and eager to do anything I wanted to do. Experiencing her loss has "challenged" my theory that exercise helps every emotion. Notice I said challenged, not changed. Working out has always been my "go to" for release of it all, until I experienced sadness.

I've learned sadness is no joke. Experiencing the absence of my dog has been debilitating. It has taken the spark out of my motivation. I thought the definition for debilitating was spot on for the way it feels. Debilitating is defined as "in a very weakened and infirm state; to make (someone) weak and infirm; hinder, delay, or weaken."

This debilitating state has made me think about others not being motivated by emotion to exercise. Experiencing trauma and tragedy myself, I've always turned to exercise for a release with little understanding why people wouldn't want the same. Now, I have a newfound grace and compassion. Healing takes time.

How do you create or get your thunder back? It's not an easy task, but it's possible. Sadness must be dealt with so it won't consume your future. So, today I'm dealing and exercising. I encourage you to work through sadness one step at a time. Exercise can be one of the best healers as you deal with loss.

Got Fitness?
Day 272

Do you remember the "Got Milk" advertising campaign that encouraged the consumption of milk for all its healthy benefits? I find that drinking milk after a run provides a good balance of carbohydrates and proteins. It, furthermore, helps repair muscles quickly and replenishes our depleted stores of glycogen. The same is true for fitness.

Fitness is an essential part of our overall health that can't be ignored. I compare it to a bicycle wheel with fitness as the hub component of the wheel. Your overall health and wellness needs to be moving forward in constant motion like a bicycle wheel in order to roll along and travel smoothly.

There's a saying, "Abs are made in the kitchen." Well, that statement is true. What we eat definitely determines how we feel, look, and even act. Continuing with the bicycle wheel analogy, what we eat are the spokes of our wheel, and there are many spokes in a bicycle wheel. Each individual spoke must be looked at as our food choices. The spokes allow stiffness in the wheel, making the wheel more efficient when spinning. A good, clean diet makes our bodies more efficient and effective as we go forward in our personal health and wellness journeys.

The fitness hub may be small, but it is a mighty part of our journeys. The hub is the central part of the bicycle wheel. It connects to the axle and the spokes. Without a hub, the bicycle wheel can't move forward effectively. The same is true with fitness. It is necessary to successfully propel us ahead.

Got fitness? You definitely need it! So I challenge you to make sure you do.

Can You Speed up Recovery Time?
Day 273

rest day   I'm not a big drinker, but I must say in my lifetime I've had too much to drink. Do you know the remedy for a hangover? TIME.

Time is also the remedy to a hardcore workout. It takes time to recover from a workout. Whether you're training for a specific event or are a fitness enthusiast who loves a challenge, it's important to know that time spent resting and recovering is just as important as the time you spend pushing yourself physically.

Here are some key areas to focus on as you take time off to recover.

Rehydrate. Staying properly hydrated helps with faster recovery, because losing as little as 2% of one's body weight through sweat can have a negative effect on exercise performance.

Fuel for a faster recovery. It matters what you are eating! The most important window for replenishing glycogen (sugars) is the four to five hours immediately after a vigorous exercise session.

Sleep. Besides scheduling regular rest days from exercise, sleep also plays a crucial role in your body's ability to bounce back from the stress of working out and becoming stronger. The exact amount of sleep needed for optimal workout recovery will vary for every exerciser, depending on age, lifestyle, and workout intensity.

Keep moving (with moderation). Although it's tempting to "veg out" after a hard workout, research has found that participating in active recovery, meaning engaging in easy, low-intensity activity the day or two after a workout, helps reduce blood lactate levels and muscle soreness more quickly than being sedentary.

It's a must to give yourself time to recover and to utilize your time wisely. You can't really speed up your recovery time, but you can do your body good by how you recover. Treat it right! :)

An Apple a Day Keeps the Doctor Away
Day 274

Proper nutrition is a good medicine. The old saying, "An apple a day keeps the doctor away," can boost your immune system when applied literally.

Almost every year you hear this cold and flu season is predicted to be a doozy. You're cautioned to be proactive to fight against germs. The best weapons in germ warfare are adequate sleep, regular exercise, and appropriate hand washing. Let's not stop there. Here are some all-natural immune "booster shot" budget-friendly foods.

Sweet potatoes: Work double duty when it comes to fighting off infection. They're filled with beta-carotene, a powerful antioxidant that transforms into vitamin A.

Grapefruit. An excellent source of vitamin C, an antioxidant shown to attack free radicals and fight infection.

Almonds. Contain healthy omega-3 fats, as well as vitamin E, the fat-soluble vitamin that protects cells against oxidation and damage. Strong, healthy cells are definitely a boost to your immune system and can help your body defend itself against germs.

Yogurt. Friendly for your gastrointestinal system—a key player in a healthy immune system. Your gut houses 25% of the immune cells in your body and provides 50% of your immune response. Plus, it's home to more than 100 trillion helpful bacteria (also called probiotics).

Garlic. Adds amazing flavor to your foods, but also gives your body allicin, an infection-fighting antioxidant that's been shown to help prevent cold and flu symptoms.

Broccoli. An excellent source of foliate, which plays an essential role in making new body cells, especially lymphocytes that search out and destroy harmful germs that invade your body.

Let's stay healthy this flu and cold season. Feeding your body good medicine along the way can never hurt. Who knew? You can give yourself an all-natural booster shot!

Environment Matters!
Day 275

If you've been on your fitness journey for very long, you should know you're going against the grain of all advertisement. Social media, billboards, restaurants, malls, even the perfect bodies you see everywhere you go, give a very confusing message. You have pressure to look perfect while eating celery or taking magic diet pills.

"What does your personal environment look like?" What do you have in your refrigerator to eat, what kind of exercise clothes do you have, what kind of shoes do you wear, what kind of friends do you have, where do you exercise, what restaurants do you go to?

These questions may seem judgmental in nature, but that's not my intent. The other morning, I was having one of those days where exercising brought dreaded feelings to mind. I was sitting in my den with a shirt and shorts on. I had to peel myself off the couch and get myself motivated somehow, someway. When I changed into my "exercise clothes" it was almost like putting on a superhero costume of motivation.

My exercise clothes were subconsciously creating an attitude for action. Soon after, I began to get excited about driving to the gym and being around like-minded friends that had similar goals. In the "Gym Environment," learning new things always occurs.

"Who are your friends?" You must have friends that have a love for fitness, too. If you only have friends that don't understand anything about exercise you probably won't get any encouragement from them to stay in the game of fitness.

Last question: "Are you willing to work on your immediate environment?" To rise out of bed daily, determined with desire to be better? What environment motivates you? I challenge you to write it down and ever loving GO FOR IT.

Do NOT Ignore Pain
Day 276

 You CANNOT ignore body pain. If you stay in the game of fitness long enough, you'll be able to decipher between exercise soreness and pain.

Exercise soreness is a normal experience caused from a good workout. Some, but not all, workouts will create Delayed Onset Muscle Soreness (DOMS). The reason this is normal is because in the process of exercise, you break down muscle and tendon tissue. The body responds by rebuilding tissue to be stronger and more productive for the next workout. There's a chemical present in this process called lactic acid, and it creates muscle soreness upon release which can resolve within a forty-eight hour rest period.

Exercise pain, on the other hand, is very different. Pain after a workout in a muscle or joint usually indicates an injury. It's brought on by a specific movement which is unlike the general soreness caused by multiple movements involved in working out. It often lasts between forty-eight hours up to a week.

The key to determining whether you're headed for a healthy soreness or an injury lies in your body consciousness—your ability to listen and identify your body's warning signs. With this basic knowledge, you can clearly identify the ways your body displays signs of fatigue or impending injury. Then you can make immediate changes to your technique to stay injury-free.

Remember to exercise in a systematic manner to work out your muscles evenly and functionally. Don't just train biceps and chest, for instance. Train opposing muscle groups to create an even pull on the joint or muscle area.

Avoiding pain during exercise is easier to control than you think. Don't ignore your pain. Instead, try to figure out what your body is telling you.

Good Pop Bad Pop
Day 277

When we place our bodies in motion, pops occur. When a client of mine experiences a pop, I usually follow up with the question, "Was that a good pop?" (did you experience some relief) or "Was it a bad pop?" (did you experience some pain).

Have you ever wondered what actually causes a pop in a joint? Popping joints can occur for any number of reasons, including normal fluid and gas in your joints, rubbing of bones or cartilage in your joints against each other, and movements of your tendons and ligaments.

While this rarely causes any pain, it can be unsettling, especially if it occurs frequently or is significant. In general, joint popping does not cause disease, is not a sign of a serious medical illness, and is not dangerous. In rare cases, however, you may need to see your doctor about it.

Popping can occur in any joint of the body. Flexing or rotating your ankle, opening and closing your hand, or moving your neck are some of the common ways this can happen. These are pops that I'd consider "Good Pops."

"Bad Pops" occur when they are accompanied by the following: pain, swelling, bruising, an obvious injury, or limited range of motion. Of course, the first thing that needs to accompany bad pops is a visit to see your physician!!

Pain is always a sign of a problem that needs treatment from a doctor. A pop in your joints should be evaluated. You should stop the exercise that caused the pop and ask yourself the question, "Was that a good pop or a bad pop?" You do not need to worry that popping will cause problems later in life. You can keep your joints healthy by exercising regularly. Our bodies were made for endless MOTION.

Physical Bodies Change With Mental Solutions
Day 278

As I sat in church this past Sunday, listening to heavenly voices, two things resonated well with my soul and have remained strong with me during the week. The two takeaways were,"There will be unexpected interruptions in life regardless of how well we plan," and "we've got to rise up and take our victory." How do we apply these two faith statements to fitness? We've got to have the right mental solutions to maintain physical change.

What is a mental solution for physical change? Awareness: being aware of what you're thinking. Do you have a victory mindset? Most of us don't. Victory with our exercise or right eating choices doesn't just fall into our laps. We've got to rise up and take our victory. This begins first with how and what you're thinking. As I've kept fitness a big part of my life, I've had to make sure my thinking is right.

I would have given up a long time ago if I hadn't set my mind to doing whatever it takes to stay fit. My routine is completely different today than it was five years ago. I can't allow myself to dwell on how much less I'm capable of today. I would drown in my incapabilities.

It doesn't matter what your age, weight, limitation, genetic pool, etc. is. Exercising will bring about a better version of YOU. I challenge you to start believing that something good can happen to you right now, no matter what your past or present looks like. We must eliminate a "give-up-easily" attitude.

I encourage you to take some time to write down a vision of fitness you'd like for yourself. Dare to ask yourself what you have been believing lately. Turn your negatives into positives; believe you can do it.

Against All Odds
Day 279

Many of our life events are beyond our control. Things just happen sometimes. No one plans to have a car accident or a fall that will leave them with life-altering physical injuries. No one plans on having herniated discs or broken bones. No one plans on events that leave them with physical limitations.

However, when life has dealt you a bad hand, I'd like to encourage you to go against all odds. Instead of giving up and giving in to the hand you have been dealt, choose to give exercise a chance. This choice may be the very thing that gives you a new lease on life.

I'm proud to share, I have a real testimony about a client who overcame physical limitations. My client's fitness journey began in a chair. Their physical limitations due to injury would only allow their exercises to be performed from a chair. What life didn't count on was this client possessed a never-give-up and a never-give-in attitude which gave them the ability to overcome every seemingly impossible limitation. Due to their decision to work out against all odds, they are now using the treadmill at an amazing pace and the free weights and resistance machines like a seasoned fitness enthusiast.

So here's the bottom line: don't let your life events keep you from pursing a new journey of health and wellness. Use whatever works against you to propel you beyond what you ever thought possible and to be the best you can be at this particular time in your life. Don't let anything get in your way. I challenge you to do as this client did and use your obstacles as opportunities to defy all odds.

Be Transformed by the 20% Rule
Day 280

rest day

Eighty percent of a formula results in an incomplete outcome. We often talk about the eighty percent of fitness being nutrition, but today, I'm most excited to present the remaining twenty percent of the formula. This twenty percent will transform your life.

Most people can diet down to their ideal weight by alternating their food choices, but to be the best you can be, exercise must be included. Exercise will not only assist in altering the size of your body, it will also tone your muscles, giving your body the shape you desire.

Exercise is a gift, not a chore. Most people dread the aspect of movement, getting sweaty, and the feeling of an elevated heart rate. With all these factors of movement comes great benefits. To name a few: high blood pressure reduction, cholesterol lowered, ideal weight management, and even irritability is counteracted. For these reasons alone, you can't afford to omit exercise from your overall health.

The beauty of the 20% is that it doesn't take much time within your twenty-four hour day. I challenge you to make the time to practice the gift of exercise. You'll surely experience your own personal transformation.

Health is a Blessing
Day 281

There are lots of things we take for granted. I don't say that to make anyone feel bad, it's simply human nature. One of the biggest things we take for granted is our mobility. Having the choice to live how we want to live is a blessing. We physically have freedom to do exactly what we want to do, and yet we don't because we're stuck focusing on what we don't like about ourselves.

My pastor shared in church one day that having good physical health is a gift. He referenced the scripture, Proverbs 17:22 (TPT) which says, "A joyful cheerful heart brings healing to both body and soul. But one whose heart is crushed struggles with sickness and depression." Our careful thoughts and actions can keep us in the blessings of good health.

We must be careful with negative thinking, because the way we think and feel often leads to action. For example, if we try on clothing that makes us feel good, our next action is to buy the clothes. That feeling led to a purchase. If we think about a particular food before we eat, we will probably eat that food. Again, our thoughts led to action.

Negative thoughts about ourselves can keep us from enjoying our lives. For instance, we might skip an event because of how we look or for fear we'd run into someone who might also see us this way. That's not how we live our best lives.

Don't get stuck thinking the wrong things about yourself. Change your negative thoughts into positive ones. Take time to be thankful for the simple things in life.

Let's rise up every morning feeling thankful for our good health. We must never take our bodies for granted. They are God-given blessings.

It is a MUST to Make Room
Day 282

Think about the word "success." How do you define success? I looked it up. The definition is: the favorable or prosperous termination of attempts; the accomplishment of one's goals; a performance or achievement that is marked by success; a person or thing that has had success, as measured by attainment of goals.

When we begin anything, especially in fitness, we want success. Right? There's a golden rule personal trainers, like myself, teach their clients who want health and wellness success. It's the F.I.T. acronym; Frequency, Intensity, and Time.

I pulled three words from the above definition of success and put them alongside the F.I.T. acronym in hopes to help you succeed in fitness. Let's consider how the words 'attempts, performance, and measured' combine with F.I.T. to create a successful fitness plan.

FREQUENCY teamed with ATTEMPTS: Successful frequency is to exercise most days in a week's span, which is 4-6 days. This means we should make room for all kinds of attempts to exercise until a favorable termination of our attempts accomplishes the goal at hand.

INTENSITY teamed with PERFORMANCE: Successful intensity is intensity during your workout either being moderate for a minimum of thirty minutes, five days a week, or vigorous for a minimum of twenty minutes, three days a week. Choose your level of performance.

TIME teamed with MEASURED: Successful time is 150 minutes weekly of aerobic exercise and 40 minutes weekly of resistance training. Get out your calendar, measure your days and time, and be sure to schedule exercise, just like you would schedule an important meeting.

I challenge you to take one simple step and declare it a MUST to make room for your fitness. Now you've got a fitness plan for success.

Shoulders Back, Guts In
Day 283

Exercisers and non-exercisers alike should constantly be reminded to keep their shoulders back and guts in. Did you know that posture ranks right up at the top of the list when talking about good health? Good posture is as important as eating right, exercising, and getting a good night's sleep.

Good posture allows you to do things with more energy and less stress/fatigue. Without good posture, it's hard to reach your full potential in becoming physically fit. Surprised? Well, you're not alone. In fact, the benefits of good posture may be among the best kept secrets. Some health problems can be avoided by improving bad posture. Good posture keeps bones properly aligned so that your muscles, joints, and ligaments work as nature intended. It gives your vital organs a proper position so they can function at peak efficiency.

Good posture helps contribute to the normal functioning of the nervous system. A person who has poor posture may often be tired or unable to work efficiently or move properly. A good example of this is sitting and working at a computer all day. Our bodies are not designed to sit in a crunched position.

Good posture naturally enables you to breathe properly. When you are breathing properly, you increase your thinking ability. People with good postures look smarter and more attractive. It's true. When you have good posture, it helps to make you feel more confident without even doing anything else differently.

Look around for yourself and see. So, I say shoulders back and guts in. It matters. I challenge you to take the time to hold yourself upright. Take the time to give your body a break from sitting. Get up and move and maintain good posture. Shoulders back and guts in; your body will thank you.

Variety Required
Day 284

Variety is required to achieve any fitness success. If you're beginning a regular exercise routine, just getting started is considered variety in itself; therefore, making the choice to exercise will immediately produce results.

But, if you work out regularly, it's easy to fall into the habit of doing the same old sets, reps, and particular exercises every time. This might make your workouts feel more comfortable, but this comfort comes at a cost. Variety is a must.

A fitness plateau will occur if variety is not implemented. To maintain a healthy and challenging exercise regimen, it's important to diversify your workouts. This is accomplished by covering the five main elements of fitness: aerobic exercise, strength training, core exercises, balance training, and stretching.

Aerobic Exercise includes any type of endurance activity that increases your heart rate for a prolonged period of time. You breathe faster, maximizing the oxygen level in your blood and using your large muscle groups.

Strength training (also known as resistance exercises) includes weights that give your muscles something to work against. Over time, your muscles adapt to that stimulus. To continue to strengthen your muscles, you need to introduce stimuli that are progressively more challenging.

Core Exercises. You may not achieve complete fitness if you just focus on aerobic exercise and strength training that only targets your arms and legs. Core exercises work the muscles in your stomach, pelvis, and lower back.

Balance is a component of fitness that people overlook. As you age, proper balance becomes increasingly important. Without good balance, you're less likely to fall or become injured.

Stretching and other flexibility exercises are cornerstones of a complete fitness routine. If you lack flexibility, your range of motion will be limited.

I challenge you to add variety to include all five elements to your training.

What are Your Triggers?
Day 285

When it comes to the way we view our own bodies and the way we look, I think it's safe to say most of us don't view ourselves very highly. The way we perceive how we look can affect many things. To change our thinking, we must be aware of our triggers.

We all have certain triggers that begin thought waves of negativity, discouragement, and hopelessness. These triggers affect our actions which can either be better or detrimental to our health. It's good to learn what triggers us, because they can lead to self-sabotage.

I'll use my own triggers as examples.

The Scale: I've learned over the years that stepping on the scale is a trigger. If I've lost weight when I step on the scale, I'm triggered to eat out of joy. If I've gained weight, I fall into a black hole of depression. Then what do I do? I eat. Now I avoid these triggers and only step on the scale for my annual check-up.

Insecurity: This is a trigger that haunts me daily. I battle insecure thoughts which can almost keep me out of the game of life. I've learned, however, to recognize certain thoughts and replace them with the Word of God. Then I pick up my boot straps and go out into this world focusing on helping others.

I challenge you to figure out your triggers and stay far away from them. Don't let them sabotage you. Learn to be content and comfortable in your own skin.

Green Tea Benefits
Day 286

Some people say green tea is the healthiest beverage on the planet. My daily goal is to drink half my body weight "in" ounces of water. But I don't argue that green tea is loaded with antioxidants and various substances that are beneficial for health.

Green tea can increase fat burning and help you lose weight. It's said that the fat-burning magic is in the highly concentrated EGCG catechin. Catechins really get the attention of the bodybuilder community. Some bodybuilders say that drinking green tea is vital for every bodybuilder trying to get ripped.

The reason for this is that green tea consumption targets fat cells and breaks down more fat, which is released into the bloodstream and becomes available for use as energy by cells that need it, like muscle cells. That's pretty cool information, even for the non-bodybuilder.

What other benefits are there to drinking green tea?

*Biological benefits. When you drink a cup of green tea, you're actually getting a large amount of substances that can reduce the formation of free radicals in the body.

*Caffeine. I know there is a lot of controversy around caffeine consumption. Green tea is known for the benefit of having caffeine. A cup of green tea contains much less caffeine (24-40 mg) than a cup of coffee (100-200 mg), but still enough to have positive effects.

*Antioxidants. Green tea has a massive range of antioxidants.

I challenge you to learn all you can about your own body. You may love green tea. You may hate green tea. I encourage you to continue seeking new things. You never know what you might discover.

Dare to Do More
Day 287

rest day

If you desire a healthier lifestyle, a great way to begin is to move. Simple tasks of movement go a long way. When you seek out ways to become a better you, it's so easy to get overwhelmed by everything you read or watch. Keeping things easy and doable, like basic movement, sets you up for results. If you're wondering what basic movement is exactly, I have some suggestions.

- Do 10 minutes of vigorous house cleaning.
- Find something productive to do in the outdoor elements. Extreme cold or hot weather makes your heart work harder, so working outside is twice as intense.
- Make fitness friends. You can never have enough friends. Make sure you have your fitness friends in your circle so you can call them up to exercise with you.
- If you've been walking and feel the need for more, the answer is still movement. Try mixing in a little jogging or running during your walking routine.
- Think you've done all you can, do 10% more.

I leave you today with the challenge to seize every opportunity for movement. Make up your mind to have an attitude to do more. Look at ways to increase movement in your daily routine: sit less, walk instead of drive, or choose more physically challenging ways to get around, such as taking the stairs instead of the elevator.

Dare to do more to be a healthier you. When the day is done, you'll be glad you did!

What Are You Magnifying?
Day 288

My church had a conference, and once again, I love relating faith to exercise. The conference theme was simple. Every action begins with a thought. Faith and exercise are the same in believing all things are possible. The scriptures say nothing is too hard for GOD. I'm thankful we can look to a GOD for all things being possible. The common desire for fitness is we want to be fit and look and feel our best.

What are you magnifying? Are you magnifying your imperfections, your last meal that was very unhealthy, your scale weight, thinking you can't do it, or never looking like you desire? You can turn your seemingly impossible situations to possibilities, like losing 100 pounds, overcoming health complications, or managing body pain. Your fitness journey will succeed or fail depending on what you are magnifying.

You must stop magnifying the wrong things, because it truly matters. You must listen to your inner dialogue and correct it if need be.

Examples:

Taking action (one exercise class/one good meal) always produces results, no matter how you feel or look on the outside.

Replace your critical view of yourself with thanksgiving for being mobile and having freedom of movement.

Tell yourself you ARE doing something NOW, not putting it off until tomorrow.

Find a positive about yourself and stay there. Tell yourself you're a work in progress and do NOT allow yourself to have a pity party or dwell on what you can't do.

Be determined to be patient as your results manifest. Believe they ARE coming.

I leave you with the question: what are you magnifying? I challenge you to constantly be aware of your inner dialogue.

Muscle Magic
Day 289

Regardless of what the late-night infomercials may say, there is really only one tried and true "magic pill" when it comes to losing weight and/or getting fit. The best news is we don't have to buy a thing to experience the magic. The magic is already within our grasp. What's the magic? It's muscle.

Yes, the magic is in our muscles. There are a couple of things in the world of weight loss that will never change:

- One pound equals 3500 calories.
- Our bodies have to realize a caloric reduction to lose weight which can be accomplished by either eating fewer calories each day and/or building muscle that will burn the calories we take in.

It has been proven over and over lean muscle mass burns calories. With each pound of muscle, the body is capable of burning up to fifty additional calories just to maintain itself. Plus, putting on just five to ten pounds of lean muscle mass will rev up your resting metabolism which is the number of calories our bodies burns to maintain life. So, simply by maintaining more muscle mass, we can roughly burn one hundred calories each and every day. This is great news particularly for those of us who struggle to reduce our daily caloric intake.

So how do we gain muscle? We gain muscle by exercising on a consistent basis. If you're exercising consistently already, keep up the good work. Great results are forecasted for your future. If you're struggling to fit exercise in your daily routine, I want to encourage you that it is never too late to get going. Tune in and exercise with me. We need each other in this lifelong fitness journey.

All Fit
Day 290

When you think about exercising, do you picture a certain type of person? Do you think that exercise isn't really your thing, but it's perfect for that certain type of person who comes to your mind?

If you answered "yes" to these questions, you're WRONG. Exercise is for every person. Whether you're tall, short, thin, wide, in good health, or in bad health, movement is exactly what a body needs. We ALL have a need for exercise. Let there be no mistake—exercise is for YOU!

Whether you're a beginner or an advanced exerciser, walking is great cardiovascular exercise. For the beginning exerciser, walking can count as your weekly exercise routine. As for the advanced exerciser, walking is great active rest. No equipment is required, just a good pair of shoes.

If you're a beginning exerciser who is excited about walking… GOOD. Start by checking with your doctor to make sure walking is right for you, then begin walking five to ten minutes at a time and gradually increase it to thirty minutes per session.

If you're an advanced exerciser, did you know that your weekly hardcore exercise regime has best results when added with active rest? Walking is considered great active rest.

Interval training is for both the beginner and the exercise veteran. It's done by varying your pace throughout your exercise session. The more power your aerobic system has, the more capacity you have to burn calories. So whether you are a walker or a marathon runner, adding interval training to your cardiovascular workout will boost your fitness.

Finally, strength training with weights is used to build muscle. This strength helps you perform daily tasks better.

Don't neglect your fitness. Our bodies NEED fitness to function properly. So come on, let's get fit!

The Overeating Struggle is Real
Day 291

Have you ever surfed the internet, read the latest and greatest food fad articles, or talked to your friends in search of those perfect ways to NOT overeat? I have! Good food … bad food, I pretty much love it all.

I have to constantly set goals for myself to find ways to keep healthy habits in front of me to keep myself in check. Today, I'd like to share some tips I find helpful:

Serve yourself healthy stuff first. I tell my kids all the time to eat their healthy food first and fun food second. Begin each meal with veggies and lean meats before placing those fattier foods and sides on your plate.

Beware of TV food advertisements. Advertisement is so powerful. Have you ever been lying in bed at night, watching TV, and all you see are those delicious breakfast commercials? So, first thing in the morning you can't wait to get to that drive-thru for that juicy something-something.

Use colored plates. The color of your dishes might make a difference in how much food you serve yourself. My mom is an interior designer and color is a powerful tool. Consider using plates in a different hue and take the time to make your food presentation a pretty one.

Hit the pause button before giving over to a craving. Pause and ask yourself the questions, "Am I bored? Am I tired? Am I stressed?" All these emotions can make you tense and make you feel out of control.

Always order the small size. A large container can tempt you to eat more food, even if you're full or it doesn't taste good.

Eat slowly. Take smaller bites. Chew your food slowly. Drink water during your meal.

We must remember every small positive choice matters.

How Clean Is Your Machine?
Day 292

What kind of car do you have? Do you like your car? Whether you like your car or not, I think we'd agree that we want our cars to be reliable. And of course, the same goes for our bodies. We need our bodies moving properly and digesting food properly, so we can go about our day properly.

Right off the bat, you may think the key to keeping your digestive tract moving properly is to eat vegetables, vegetables, and more vegetables! Well, you're right! Eating vegetables is a good answer. Whether you eat vegetables or not, I have an interesting fact to share. Typically an individual holds up to seven meals in their digestive tract. That is why it is extremely important to make sure your digestive tract is moving properly.

This fact poses the question of what kind of fuel do you put in your car? Is it regular, super, or premium fuel? We should categorize our food the same way. Raw food is like premium fuel. Raw foods act as quality roughage. For example, eat anything you can in raw form, like raw vegetables, nuts, seeds, sprouted foods, or legumes. Feeding your body the roughage it needs will keep the typical seven meals moving properly through your digestive tract.

We need to make sure our bodies are running at high performance and clog-free. The right amount of roughage keeps our "engine" clean and running for miles and miles, just like our car runs best at high performance with high octane fuel.

To conclude, let's try to make a daily effort to eat our vegetables. Frequently ask yourself the question, "How clean is my machine?" We need clean machines/bodies for our best performance in this race called life.

Determine to be Determined

rest day Never underestimate the power of determination. I say that because I have seen what it can do.

Here's a real example of how determination changed a life:

Just over 12 months ago, I walked into the gym to meet a new client. As soon as I looked in her eyes, I knew she was ready to change her life. She was not only beaming with a desire to make a change, but she also exuded a determination that I knew couldn't be stopped.

Her desire was to turn from a life of inactivity to one of activity. From that day on, she fully embraced fitness, health, and wellness. Her unwavering determination has made that a reality.

Her hard work, sweat, and 'never give up' attitude have driven her to become 80 pounds lighter and 6 sizes smaller than where she began. I can't tell you how much of an inspiration she has been and continues to be to me.

Our possibilities in life are endless. With determination and hard work, the right plan specifically designed for you will see those possibilities come to fruition.

I challenge you to believe that you can simply embrace possibility (it can happen) to the realm of probability (realizing it will happen) and on to one of victorious reality (experiencing that it did happen). You can become a better you.

Be determined to live with a purpose and a resolve to see it through. Start today to live a determined life.

Why Not to Give Up
Day 294

As I sat in church this past Sunday, I heard a wonderful message delivered by my pastor on why we should never give up. I see a lot of correlation between faith and fitness. This message made me think of the importance of keeping fitness in the forefront of our daily life and how we must pursue not giving up.

I had a former client who attended my classes for years. She grew discouraged over time because she didn't think what she was doing mattered. I watched her discouragement grow as I encouraged her to keep up the good work and told her what she was doing DID matter.

Her discouragement finally got the best of her, and she stopped coming to class. Not much time had passed before she came back, 30 pounds heavier. She realized there was a lot of good happening; what she was doing really did matter. If we give into the lie that "it's not doing me any good," we could run the risk of quitting, too. You never know all the good things that are taking place within while exercising regularly, until you stop.

I challenge you to eliminate your quit button. Find things that are exciting to keep you moving. Find one good thing; be determined to grab hold and not let go. Make the effort to find the good in your daily choices. Effort does matter and could be the very factor that keeps you in the game.

Keep your chin up and in forward motion. Don't lay down your health and wellness; remember it's gift of moving freely. Don't take your mobility for granted, and you'll quickly see that you've earned an "A" for your effort. This is a reason all the more not to give up.

Simple Says It All
Day 295

I love using acronyms to makes things simple and easy to remember. I even use the word SIMPLE as an acronym because it's a powerfully effective tool when implemented for workouts.

S is for steps, steps, and more steps. Walking, hiking, or whatever makes you happy. Stepping is my new favorite exercise. You can literally step your way to better health. You can even set your own personal goals and track them with apps on your phone.

I is for intensity. Intensity is what we need for individual growth. We each have a different intensity scale. No matter what fitness level you find yourself in, you can constantly challenge yourself. New exercises and challenges are a wonderful way to keep your intensity in check.

M is for movement. Our bodies are made to get us from point A to point B. They aren't made to sit for long, extended periods of time. They are made to MOVE. You must embrace any kind of safe movement.

P is for push. Pushing yourself brings on the good kind of pain. Laborious workouts are key for taking you to the next fitness level.

L is for Learn. Learning new things breaks the mundane. If you've exercised long enough on a regular basis, you know some boredom can set in. So, you must remain open to seeking out and doing new activities.

E is for Exercise. Exercise regularly. Exercising isn't a one-time deal. You've got to exercise on a regular basis in order to reach the maximum benefits.

These simple steps offer great gain and benefit to your body. I encourage you to keep at it, keep it simple, and never give up.

Focus
Day 296

When you begin your journey toward better health and wellness, you need a focal point. Have you ever tried to do something good for yourself, and it seems like everything in your life falls apart to keep you from pursuing your personal goals? This journey is no easy task, and life's storms are guaranteed to come.

It's a must to stay focused. Make it a weekly priority to exercise 20 to 30 minutes two or three times a week no matter what, but don't expect perfection. Perfectionists feel the need to do their full exact fitness routine or do nothing at all. Aiming to be perfect with your fitness can lead to giving up when things aren't perfect, like missing a day or two.

Focus on convenience. Do whatever you can to remove obstacles to exercise. Make it as convenient as possible. If you are time-pressed, don't spend 30 minutes driving to a gym. Try exercising at home to fitness videos. If you're too tired to work out at the end of the day, it may be more convenient to exercise in the morning.

The right focus could be the very ingredient that you need to catapult yourself into the shape you've only dreamt about. There is a scripture I love to focus on. A part of Philippians 4:8 says to think upon true things, just things, "whatever things are of GOOD REPORT," if there is anything praiseworthy meditate upon these. Make sure to stay "good" focused.

If you're putting forth any effort to better your health and wellness… it's a GOOD REPORT. I challenge you to find good and keep it your focus. I guarantee more good will come. There are so many rewards and benefits just waiting to be developed within you.

Temptation or Temptations?
Day 297

Temptation is generally defined as something that can persuade or lure us away from what we know to be right. But did you know, there are two types of temptation? If we fail to recognize the temptations threatening our fitness plans, we may derail our quest to reach our fitness goals.

The first type of temptation is based on outward or external circumstances. For instance, we may be tempted to put off our workout because we have to take our children somewhere, go to the grocery store, attend a meeting, or go to work. Early morning workouts can often circumvent possible external temptations or events that may keep us from working out most days.

The other type of temptation is inward or internal. This type of temptation involves our minds and our emotions which can create a stronghold in our lives if we don't break its grip. Internal temptations tell us things like: we'll never change because we have always been that way; we ate too much to work it off; or we just can't do it. Hear me when I say it's time to stop repeating these lies, because if we don't, we will eventually believe them.

I'm here to tell you, it's time to change. Become aware of these two types of temptations in your life so you can plan different, act different, and become different. Look ahead and not behind. The past is who you were, not who you are, or who you are going to be. Put forth the effort to reduce or eliminate these daily temptations in your life so you can successfully meet your fitness goals.

The Perfect Diet
Day 298

There is a tailor-made diet to be discovered for each of us. The part most of us don't understand is it has to be discovered. Although it may take much trial and error, there is an eating plan that will work perfectly for you. Each diet needs a basic structure, including proteins, vegetables, complex carbohydrates, and fruits.

Write a list of the food groups you like most. After you've discovered your own unique "favorite list," this basic structure can catapult you into your own unique food plan. The next thing to figure out is the personal food combinations that work best for you. It's really simple to figure this out. Let your body be your guide. At your next meal, eat your personalized proteins, carbohydrates, fruits, and vegetables; take note of how you feel afterward.

Do you feel energized or tired? Some foods may leave you feeling bloated or sluggish. You may even suffer from indigestion. On the other hand, you may feel great and have extra energy.

Figure out the best times of the day to eat. Then decide how you'd like to consume your calories. For example, you could eat small meals like split breakfasts, split lunches, and a very light dinner. This gives you a total of 5 small meals to meet your caloric intake for the day. In return, you'll get a maximum amount of energy. It's a win-win.

You've got to enjoy life. We all love our vices, like cakes, chips, cookies, fatty meats, adult beverage, or pies. These foods have their place. Add them into your weekly eating plan. Plan ahead for these days. It IS possible to find the perfect diet on which your body best thrives. Learn all you can.

Fitness is a Relationship
Day 299

Have you ever thought of comparing exercise to a relationship? Cultivating a good relationship takes time and energy as does exercise. A good relationship with no time invested will fizzle out and become a distant acquaintance. Little time invested in exercise will fizzle quickly too.

Attitude also has a lot to do with longevity of exercise. Just like in our relationships, no one wants to be around someone with a sour-puss attitude. A weekly fitness routine should be approached with a good attitude—like your attitude when you're with someone you enjoy being around.

When you want to hang out with friends, what do you do? You schedule a time to get together. The same is true for exercise. Schedule a regular workout time and do it. Some of the most committed exercisers do it every day. Sit down with your weekly schedule and build in an hour each day. Be good to your body just like it's a trusted friend.

Do you spend time with your friends because you have to? Of course not. Do you exercise out of guilt, self-disgust, or fear? You shouldn't. When you spend time with loved ones, it's fun to do exciting and adventurous things together. Exercise should be looked at as an adventure too.

When you're planning for the week, make room for some variety. Think fun and creatively. By nature, humans need change and variety to stay motivated.

How is your fitness relationship? Is it good or can it use some fine-tuning? No matter where you are in your fitness, I'm sure you can find something that needs some adjusting. We're all a work in progress so don't beat yourself up. When we invest time in people and in ourselves, we'll always reap a harvest.

The Prerequisite of All Fitness Success
Day 300

rest day The prerequisite to any health and wellness success is a determination to accomplish what you've set out to do. Fitness success is not for the weak at heart. You have to set your sails forward and be determined not to give up or give in. Hang on to your vision, beginning with your first decision to make a change.

At first, the scale might not move, but other positive things are transpiring. For instance, you have to buy new pants or your energy levels are better than they've been in years. You never know what your initial victories will look like. Make sure to take notice and rejoice. Be aware not to set the wrong type of expectations.

Be open to any positive responses. Allow those positives to be your focal point and motivator. The problem is most people soon lose sight of any positive outcome and quit. Believing you can't do it makes you settle with your present fitness, completely defying the abundant results that are coming your way.

Be determined to press forward as you glance over your shoulder to see just where NOT quitting has carried you. Results may take longer than you imagined, maybe even years. That's not a bad thing. Exercise is like eating your next meal. It must become a part of your survival.

There are so many rewards that come with a committed life of exercise. What doesn't challenge you won't change you. Take on a challenge today. There's NO time to think about the "what ifs" or the "I can'ts." There's work to be done, such as working out to my exercise videos and eating good food. Most importantly, strive for good health and wellness.

Walk On
Day 301

rest day

The super busy season is coming up on us. My advice to you is, don't stop; walk on. The super snacks season is coming up on us. My advice to you is, don't stop; walk on.

The holiday season is just around the corner, beginning with Halloween, and it doesn't end until January 2nd. Snacks and parties will be abundant, in addition to the temptation to slow down or even stop exercising.

I challenge you to continue walking on; don't stop and be tempted to follow in the footsteps of many of the exercising population who will allow their temptations to completely derail all their fitness plans, hard work, and success.

If you stop now in your fitness journey, when January rolls around you'll wish you didn't stop. When you're ready to start back up again, it will be much harder than if you kept your exercise routine intact.

January is not the time to think about losing weight; the time is now. Resolve the matter of it even being a consideration to quit but instead consider it a time to lose, maintain, and not regain your weight.

Be determined today to not stop. Walk on and keep up with your fitness. Trust me, you'll be glad you did!

Winter Fitness Check List
Day 302

When the days get shorter and cooler, it is more important than ever to pre-plan your daily exercise goals so you can reach them. I've done this for years, and it really works.

Below are a few suggestions and practical steps that have worked well for me.

- Lay out appropriate exercise clothing (warm-up suit, fitness shoes, socks, etc.) the night before.
- Pack your workout bag the night before.
- Don't forget your towel and be sure to go ahead and fill your water bottle in advance.
- Determine in advance what time you will exercise and commit to keeping it.
- Treat this appointment with the same level of importance as any other appointment you schedule in your day.
- Don't go on emotion. Exercise in your allotted time no matter how you feel at the time.
- Make sure you keep variety in your workouts.

During colder months, we are typically home more often, so you might include your family in your workout plans. You may also include your friends on occasion, but don't depend on them to always be your motivator.

The change of seasons can really get us off track especially when we don't like cold weather. I encourage you to embrace the change in seasons and don't lose your momentum! You won't be sorry.

Movement is a Must
Day 303

Movement beyond your allotted exercise time is vital to the success of your health and wellness. The movement that I'm talking about is movement outside of your scheduled "exercise sessions." For maximum results, there is an acronym I'd like to share: F.I.T.

Our "exercise sessions" should consist of frequency, intensity, and time (F.I.T.). These are the three vital components needed to produce results. Frequency is following a structured workout at a gym, home, or a group class, done 5 days a week. Intensity consists of challenging exercise sessions followed by recovery sessions. Time is both frequency and intensity lasting 30 or 60 minutes for each session. You'd think these exercise sessions would be all we need, but think again.

An overlooked piece of fitness is an active lifestyle. What is an active lifestyle? It's what you do during your daily spare time. Active living generally means adding some form of physical activity to your leisure time. This is defined by simply doing activities that you like to do, whether it's skiing, playing your favorite sport, fishing, or diving. As long as there is some movement involved, it's considered an active lifestyle.

What is considered an inactive lifestyle? Filling your spare time with things that require sitting. For example: reading, knitting, watching movies, or completing crossword puzzles. Now these things aren't bad! I love to read or binge watch movies myself. I have to strategically plan outdoor/indoor fun activities that require movement.

I encourage you to evaluate how you spend your spare time. I'll bet you haven't given much thought to your spare time before, especially if you're an avid exerciser. Movement is a must! You'll be so glad you did.

Don't Get Tricked by Grabbing for the Treats
Day 304

Put up your dukes and keep yourself protected. The annual holiday quadruple threat is here: Halloween, Thanksgiving, Christmas, and New Year's. While the treats during these holidays are great, the terrible tricks they play on your already achieved health and wellness gains can be brutal.

Now, in particular, is the time to stay on guard in your fitness walk. Through the next few months, every single bit of exercise you squeeze in and every good food choice you make will help you to emerge from the holidays a healthy victor.

Our goal through the holidays is to maintain what we have achieved and not to regain. As a result of your diligence, when the first of the year rolls around, you'll be many steps ahead. The answer to staying ahead is to say NO to a number of things.

Say NO to sitting down with or without your kids and ravaging through their Halloween treats. Say NO to those office goodies that always show up during the holidays. Most of all, say NO to giving up and convincing yourself you'll just worry about it after the first of the year.

Saying YES to fitness and healthy food choices is how you will win this fight. So, I challenge you to say YES to taking a walk. YES to visiting a gym with a friend. YES to participating in one of my video classes. YES to skipping a meal simply because you aren't hungry.

I encourage you to keep your guard up and watch out for that sucker punch of temptation that will try to knock you off your fitness journey. Treat yourself to a YES today.

Staying Fit Through the Holidays
Day 305

 November and December can be overwhelmingly busy. The truth of the matter is, most people do not keep their normal weekly fitness obligations. There's still a way to implement fitness into your schedule. If you say, "There's no way," well, I say right back, "Oh yes there is a way." I have two suggestions that are quick and effective. If you can stick to one of these particular methods, you'll be better protected against holiday weight gain and more ready and able to work toward your New Year's resolution without feeling too far gone.

Focus on Strength Workouts: For this particular quick and effective workout, you'll only need a barbell and weight plates or dumbbells. Your goal is to do one set of 6 to 8 reps, utilizing power movements like: Barbell/dumbbell squats, Barbell/dumbbell deadlift, Barbell/dumbbell bent over rows, Barbell/dumbbell shoulder presses, Barbell/dumbbell bicep curls, Barbell/dumbbell stationary lunges, etc. Each of these exercises need a rest interval for 30-60 seconds (example: in place jog). You need to push these single sets to your limits, but with wisdom and safety, of course.

Focus on Core Workouts: This workout is meant to help improve your core strength. Best choice is if you have access to a stability ball, BOSU Ball, or weight bench. Pick two particular core-related exercises, like a light dumbbell chest press and an abdominal exercise, performing both exercises on a stability ball. Do each exercise in a superset form (meaning the chest exercise and abdominal exercise done with no rest), then rest for 30 seconds between supersets. It'll challenge your abdominal wall and balance.

Remember, these two focused training workouts are quick but effective and doable. You can still work out successfully. Bring on the holidays with much excitement and joy.

It's a Simple Decision
Day 306

Having the holidays on our heels, I thought it would be most appropriate to talk about fitness and nutrition choices we make over the next couple of months.

Our lives are made up of decisions that bring about future events. Usually an event takes place due to a past decision we've made. If you study for an upcoming exam, the outcome equals good grades. If you decide to do home improvements, the outcome equals a beautiful home.

It's the same with your health and wellness decisions. If you decide to exercise, the outcome equals better health. If you decide to eat right, the outcome equals guaranteed results. Goals, desires, and dreams are all based on what you decide to do today that equals future events.

Simple decisions that equal a good outcome:

Say NO to soda. Soft drinks consumed each day can increase your risk of being overweight by 65 percent. Instead, sip plain or sparkling water with lemon added for flavor.

Eat like clockwork. When you're not hungry, you're less tempted by fun foods.

Pack in the protein. Make sure you've had your protein at every meal. The digestion of protein involves a longer process than the digestion of carbohydrates, therefore keeping you full longer.

K.I.S.S. (Keep it Simple Sweetheart). Basic staple foods such as lean proteins like chicken, turkey, eggs, and fish; salads with 1 tablespoon of dressing; apples with almond or peanut butters. Avoiding sauces and condiments keeps your food simple and equals less calories.

These next couple of months are full of blessing. I challenge to keep clean eating and your exercise daily on point. Let's make the decisions now to do the simple things to stay on track. You will reap an incredible outcome.

RE-FOCUS With the Basics
Day 307

| rest |
| day |

Every little step of exercise makes a big difference. Many people get discouraged and fall off the fitness wagon during these last two months of the year. So sometimes we need a back-to-the-basics reminder to help us stay with our fitness routines.

A simple way to keep you in the habit is to take a ten-minute pause to exercise most days of the week. Strive to implement movement into your day—you can walk just about anywhere! Attend a fitness class just once a week for a great benefit. Lay out your clothes the night before so you'll be more apt to go to class. Don't allow the excuse of an interrupted schedule keep you trapped in the cage of inactivity.

Taking this time to refocus on the simplicity of basic exercise is guaranteed to leave you feeling energized and encouraged. It will get you going in the right direction to tackle whatever tasks lie ahead of you. Looking back over these two months, you will see how little it took to maintain what you worked so hard to achieve throughout the year. If you stick with it, you will be amazed by your results and thankful that you took the time to exercise.

I challenge you to keep moving through the holiday season. Exercise just as you are and commit to the time you have to do it. It is possible to overcome the busy holiday schedule excuses. So stay encouraged and stay the course!

The Power of the Hip Flexors
Day 308

rest
day   Hip flexors are a pretty specific group of muscles, but they're a
      mighty group of muscles. Whether you go for speed, longevity,
or simply recreation, your hip flexors will probably get tight or even sore
at some point.

What are hip flexors? The hip flexors are a "group of muscles" that
allow you to lift your knees toward your chest and bend forward from the
hips. I believe it's really good to know a little bit about where these specific muscles are so we can better care for ourselves. My hope in sharing
these particular muscles is to help you narrow down the pain or injury to
a "specific hip flexor" so you can research how exactly to stretch and care
for yourself.

For further research, the hip flexors group consists of the *iliopsoas*,
the *rectus* femurs, the *sartorius*, the tensor *fasciae latae*, and the inner
thigh muscles, which consist of the adductor *longus*, *brevis*, *pectineus*,
and *gracilis*.

Tight hip flexors aren't just for the elite exerciser. Tight hip flexors
are a common problem among those of us who sit at a desk most of the
day. When you spend a lot of time in a seated position, the hip flexors
remain in a shortened position. This requires proper stretching to avoid
tight hip flexors or even an injury.

There are simple things you can do every day to help reduce your
risk of hip flexor pain or injury. If you sit at a desk for long periods of time,
try to get up and move around every hour or so. If you're an avid runner or even a recreational runner, warm up properly before any physical
activity and stretch regularly at the end of each workout. Your hips will
thank you for it!

Exercise-Induced Asthma
Day 309

I was talking to a client of mine (who is precious, I might add) who struggles with exercise-induced asthma. I'm not very familiar with this condition, but I have a little understanding that our oxygen levels need to be greater than 95%. Ninety-five percent is generally considered to be a normal range. On the other hand, when oxygen saturation levels fall below 92%, the pressure of the oxygen in your blood is too low to penetrate the walls of the red blood cells, and this can be very dangerous.

My daughter struggled with her breathing a couple of years ago, and not understanding the seriousness of her condition, I took her to the walk-in clinic. We soon learned that her oxygen level was at 92, and they immediately sent me to the emergency room. She was diagnosed with walking pneumonia. I'm aware she wasn't struggling with exercised-induced asthma, but you don't want to mess around with breathing. It's serious.

The definition for exercise-induced asthma (EIB) is a narrowing of the airways in the lungs that is triggered by strenuous exercise. The preferred term is exercise-induced bronchoconstriction (EIB). It causes shortness of breath, wheezing, coughing, and other symptoms during or after exercise. When you begin to exercise, you breathe faster and deeper due to the increased oxygen demands of your body. You usually inhale through your mouth, causing the air to be drier and cooler than when you breathe through your nose. The dry or cold air is the main trigger for airway narrowing (bronchoconstriction).

Asthma or no asthma, pace yourself. With effective management, people with EIB can perform and excel in a variety of fitness activities. :) The more we know about how our bodies perform, the better off we'll be!

The Painless Path
Day 310

It sure would be nice if taking the painless path really worked. We've all experienced the easy way before, but soon discovered that what does come easy won't last. What lasts, won't come easy. Our health and wellness journey is a hard journey; if you work hard, it lasts.

A very slim minority of the American population works hard to continue to keep fit. Less than 3% of Americans meet the basic qualifications for a healthy lifestyle.

A healthy lifestyle includes the following:

• Moderate exercise for 150 minutes per week or vigorous exercise for 75 minutes per week

• Body fat percentage under 20% for men and 30% for women

• No smoking

We must always embrace the narrow path of doing what we know we should do. Evaluate any trend that seems to be an easy way out. Find the fun in your healthy way of living. Surround yourself with like-minded people that eat healthy and exercise regularly.

I challenge you to resolve yourself to the fact that there is NO painless path. You WILL take the road that might seem impossible. Be determined to discover the blessing of working hard and achieving your goals. You're ready to give it 100%, knowing it'll take a lot of sweat and hard work to accomplish the task.

Remember, what comes easy won't last. What lasts, won't come easy. The FIGHT is always worth it. It ONLY produces success.

Hydration
Day 311

Keeping the body hydrated is essential. The best way to keep the body hydrated is to drink water. The foods we eat and the beverages we drink count for some water intake, but it's not enough.

Most people walk around dehydrated and they don't even know it. Everyone loses water throughout the day. It is lost through your breath, sweat, urine, etc. You lose even more fluid when you're in a hot climate. It can be a task and inconvenient to keep the body hydrated, but it's definitely worth the trouble. One of the dangers of becoming dehydrated is that your body no longer has enough fluid to transmit blood to your organs. It's a constant effort to replace lost fluid to stay healthy.

A common recommendation is to drink six to eight, 8-ounce glasses of water daily. This amount varies depending on health, exercise frequency, and how hot and dry the climate is.

The easiest way to see if you're dehydrated is by the color of your urine. If you're drinking enough water, your urine will be clear or pale yellow. A darker yellow means you aren't drinking enough water.

You can drink too much water. Water consumed in excess could dilute the amount of sodium in your body. However, it's rare that anyone drinks too much water. The risk is highest for people who do endurance sports, such as running marathons. Experts advise athletes who do intense activity to drink a sports drink that contains sodium, other electrolytes, and some sugar. The normal exerciser doesn't need sports drinks; water should be their go-to.

Water keeps every part of your body working properly. I encourage you to stay hydrated. Be aware of how much water you are actually consuming.

Embracing the Beauty
Day 312

Welcome to our microwave society. In a matter of seconds, you can have a hot meal. Type a topic into a search engine and in a jiffy you can find thousands of articles on any subject.

In many areas of our lives we've lost all concept of time. We are no longer accustomed to putting in the time that it takes to achieve excellence. Time invested eventually produces a work of distinction and beauty.

One client's testimony of how she embraced fitness and the time it takes to produce real results:

"When I realized last night the exercise segment of running wasn't as challenging to me as it had been, I was so inspired. The results I've experienced took way more time than I would've liked, but I am seeing progress. The exercise group setting really helps me not focus on the time and pain invested. I know whether I attend the class or not they'd be there anyway getting the results I'm missing. Being with others motivates me. It brings out the competitiveness in me to push myself.

I find myself on the weekends just standing in the bathroom doing squats. If I am just lying around, I try to do some abs. Playing around with my kids, I throw in some leg lifts. It has taken me a long time to drop 20 pounds, but in the process I've embraced the beauty of the journey. It's been a learning process. I don't regret any amount of time that it took for me to be where I am today."

My client's patience paid off. In addition to losing weight, her arms and mid-section are developed and her overall body is toned. She exemplifies what time and fitness can produce.

I encourage you to embrace the time it takes.

Opportunity
Day 313

When you think of the word opportunity, what comes to mind? Good things, I'm sure. The definition of opportunity is: 1. an appropriate or favorable time or occasion 2. a situation or condition favorable for attainment of a goal. Let's talk about given and created opportunities.

A given opportunity is when someone lends you their lake house for the weekend or invites you on a once in a lifetime trip with all expenses paid. Who wouldn't like a given opportunity? We should all count our blessings when we're met with such unexpected, pleasant surprises that we didn't even ask for.

As for created opportunities, they must be created. Creating healthy fitness opportunities set you up to fully enjoy the given opportunities. When it comes to our health and wellness, we must create opportunities like making the time to exercise and treating our body well. This will ensure we stay the course and on top of such a finicky topic that is constantly changing.

A sample created opportunity plan:

I will exercise Monday-Friday at 6:00 a.m. for one hour.

MONDAYS/WEDNESDAYS/FRIDAYS I will do a 30-minute cardiovascular exercise (treadmill run) followed by a 30-minute total body toning workout.

On TUESDAYS/THURSDAYS I'll do an extended cardiovascular workout of 45 minutes of cycling followed by 15 minutes of core and stretch.

I'll train at the gym before work, so my created opportunity doesn't interfere with my family time.

The next time a given opportunity comes your way, count your blessings and seize the moment. Don't let a once in a lifetime opportunity pass you by. Remember the same is true for a created opportunity. Our health and wellness is a gift that is extremely finicky. Life is a gift. I challenge you to seize all opportunities, given and created.

Happy Place
Day 314

rest day   If we could sit down and chat one-on-one, and I asked you the question, "What is your happy place," an image would come to mind. If you could go there right now, I'll bet this particular place brings peace, happiness, rest, joy, anything good, and can put any unpleasant circumstances on hold temporarily.

People in general don't associate a happy place with exercise. There's such a bad connotation with the word 'fitness.' Health and wellness are NOT happy words. Sometimes even the mention of the word 'fitness' makes people feel and think 'dread.'

I'd like to change that perspective. When you think thoughts of being in shape, it brings you to a happy place instantaneously, but then when you begin to plan action steps toward better health, questions and concerns tend to arise. Soon, you're assaulted with doubt when your first exercise class doesn't produce the immediate results you're after; thoughts of "I can't do this, what was I thinking, I'm never going to accomplish my goals, exercise isn't for me, I'm embarrassed to even think I ever could," etc....the lies continue.

I'm here to tell you, you can find a happy place in fitness. It first begins with, "Yes, I Can." We so easily get down on ourselves and quit. The self-talk of can't, never, what was I thinking … must not be entertained. It sounds so cliché, but I've watched many individuals begin all gung ho, then the negative self-talk comes in and they soon let go of the rope and quit. Self-talk is a real deal breaker.

I challenge you to find your happy place in fitness. You have one body. Exercise makes you alert, ready for action, and in a place to bless others.

Don't Resist Resistance Training
Day 315

rest day What people don't understand about a well-rounded fitness program is the resistance training aspect of fitness. It's a critical, but often ignored, facet of fitness training. Especially when it comes to females incorporating resistance training; it is needed in their workouts, too.

Implementing resistance training is what makes the difference in taking you to a new level in your health and wellness. If you want to burn fat, do resistance training. If you feel underweight and scrawny, do resistance training. If you want to lose weight, do resistance training.

If you want to be "fit," do resistance training.

Muscles are a stimulus. When you do resistance training, your muscles respond by a range of stimuli that can increase the volume of cells. In turn, your muscle grows; this is called muscle hypertrophy.

The opposite is true if you don't do resistance training. You can experience muscle atrophy. In simple terms, if you don't use your muscles you lose muscle. Whatever spectrum you come from, it's important to do resistance training.

The key is to challenge your muscles enough so that they will make a change. It doesn't have to be bone-crushing weight you lift, but it needs to be enough to provide some resistance. Whatever your fitness goal is, some of your answers will be found in resistance training. This is achieved by adding more weight or trying different exercise routines.

The challenge I'd like to leave you with today is to not resist resistance training. Not every weightlifting exercise is right for everyone. Continue to seek out the right exercise that works for you. You'll never regret the continued search for pumping up your own unique routine. With a little time, let resistance make the difference for you!

Yes I Will, No I Won't
Day 316

Choosing to exercise is not a one-time decision. In fact, it is a daily decision that is oftentimes determined by our self-talk. Think about it, more times than not the number one single thing that keeps us from exercising is us! We allow our self-talk to make that choice for ourselves.

Daily success is learning to master the art of positive self-talk. Positive self-talk has motivated many people to attend class, and many of those days are not set in the perfect atmosphere. I had one precious client that would come to class and say she was on the struggle bus and not having the best day, but she came anyway. Other excuses used to justify not exercising could include "it's really cold out," "I have 1,000 other things to do," or simply "I just don't feel like it." The truth is, we all can talk ourselves out of fitness class 100 times. The mind cycles "I'm not going, yeah I'll go, no I won't." You know, that kind of thinking all day long can be broken. When that mind cycle is broken, you are left feeling grateful afterwards, with less tension, stress, and frustrations.

Our self-talk is most significant in our fitness journey. It can turn a defeated mentality into one of victory. It can be the difference between success in reaching our fitness, health, and wellness goals or spending another day regretting that we said no.

The beautiful thing is that every day gives us another chance to not live in regret. No one said this would be easy, but I'm here to tell you it's doable. Talk to yourself and to people who can give you encouragement. Be determined to not give into defeated talk!

Reviving Your Workout is a Must
Day 317

One of my most frequent prayers about my job is to keep all my classes innovative, creative, challenging, and fun. I know the longer you maintain an exercise routine, the more important it is to keep it fresh.

We all risk choosing the couch over physical activity. Apart from maintaining workouts, adding variety is a guaranteed way to achieve better results.

Here are a few methods that will help keep things revived when you're feeling blah.

Mix and match strength-training exercises and cardio. Combine strength exercises like push-ups and squats with fast-paced cardio intervals like jump rope or a sprint.

Vary the repetitions and sets with the weight selection. If you take my classes on YouTube, an example during the rotation time is to count to 20 with a pulse at the end of each exercise.

Vary the lengths and types of your workouts. For instance, split your workout days and add high-intensity interval training (HIIT), which is a short and super intense cardiovascular session.

Experiment with different variations of one exercise. There are many different ways to do push-ups and lunges. Take a plank for example. Do a plank with a crunch, with a twist, or a side plank into a low plank.

Try different equipment. Don't be afraid to try equipment. Switch between barbells, dumbbells, kettle bells, medicine balls, resistance bands, jungle gym straps, and cables.

Work on core stability. Once you feel strong and confident performing exercises with great technique on solid ground, you can progress to other surfaces such as BOSU or stability balls to further engage and strengthen your core stabilizers.

In my home, the word "boring" is a bad word. So, if you're feeling the blahs, hang on. I challenge you to revive your workouts to keep on achieving your goals.

Holiday Reminders
Day 318

 Before you know it, we'll be in a new year. We can never have enough reminders to keep our health and wellness in check.

Today, here are some simple things to keep in the forefront of our minds.

Always plan ahead. When it comes to maintaining your diet and workout plan over Thanksgiving, Christmas, and New Year's, have your plan in play.

Improvise your workout. As holiday obligations arise, sticking to your normal workout routine can start to feel like an impossible task. Try getting up earlier and doing a short cardio/strength training session.

Avoid sitting for too long. The holidays are all about parties and visits with family and friends, but when you're not dancing at those parties or shopping with family, you might often find yourself sitting for extended amounts of time. Incorporate mall or outdoor walks. Even a quick trip to the park is a good, healthy activity.

Be party wise. I used to think I needed to starve myself before an evening dinner or party. But it's really quite the contrary. By not eating all day, you're saving calories, but you'll be far more likely to go hog wild at a party if you're starving.

Manage stress. Another "must do" for the holiday season is to learn how to better manage your stress levels. I know that's easier said than done. Exercise is a great manager of stress.

Try healthy recipes. Healthy recipes can be better than old fashioned Grandma recipes. Try finding healthy alternatives to some of your traditional holiday favorites.

It's an exciting life to be fit. I encourage you to keep your focus.

What Do Your Holiday Breaks Look Like?
Day 319

I want to encourage you to enjoy this time of year but to also make some effort to exercise and eat within some sort of boundary. These small, seemingly insignificant choices make a big difference and are worth the effort.

I'd like to share a story: I had a client who was extremely motivated. She came to me overweight, desiring to lose weight. She actively lost 1 to 2 pounds each week. She was on a 1,500-calorie per day eating plan. She exercised five times per week, burning 300 calories per session.

To create a healthy caloric deficiency for my client, she had to omit 500 calories a day from her diet. Multiply that by 7 days in a week and that equals 3,500 omitted calories. 3,500 calories is important because 3,500 calories equals 1 pound of fat. Then I added in her exercise regimen (300 calories per session, times 5 sessions), thus allowing her to continue losing weight at a healthy rate.

I challenge you to resist taking a complete break from everything related to health and wellness. Hold on to some kind of goal that will keep you active through the rest of this year. It's as simple as not eating that extra 500-calorie "something" daily. Or pack your gym bag with a determination to keep up the good work just like my client did.

It's all about that caloric deficiency. It doesn't take much to stay in shape by being aware of what your body needs for fuel and how much you consume and burn. Taking a break doesn't and shouldn't have to be an all or nothing decision. Minimizing any weight gain through exercise and practicing moderation is very possible. Making good choices will always be well worth your time.

Never Too Late to Turn it Around
Day 320

Have you ever thought you've simply gone too far and it's too late to make a change for the better? I sure have. Today, let's talk about ways to turn our health around. I'm here to tell you that it's never ever too late, no matter your weight, age, stature, or environment.

I'll never forget being in the gym in my early twenties and meeting a lady who was in her mid-fifties. She looked phenomenal. I asked her questions about her fitness and learned her secret to success. I was surprised when she told me on her 50th birthday she was sick and overweight. She said, "I was so tired of being the way I was, I decided to get off my couch and join the gym!" She shared she'd never been fit in her life until then. She felt the best she'd ever felt. If you're in your fifties and think it's too late, it's not.

My daughter studied skin anatomy in school. She learned, as humans, we molt our skin like other animals do to make room for new skin growth. If we molted like snakes we would have empty casts of ourselves lying around. But luckily, we shed skin in stages. During puberty, skin regeneration is at its quickest, but as we age the regeneration slows down. If skin is reproducing at such a rapid rate, then we too can make a big difference by how we treat our bodies. If you have a bad diet and are completely sedentary, it's not too late to make a change.

How about we work toward celebrating being healthy, focusing on our well being, and not worrying another second about our weight and exterior shell of a body? We're relational people that have movement in common; let's move together.

Finding Freedom From Excess
Day 321

rest day   We're all looking to either achieve or maintain our ideal weight.
If you're having trouble getting there or staying there, it's likely
that some excess factors may be in the way. Let's take a look and see.

Excess. As a society, we are faced with excess every single day. Dining out experiences entice us with big gulps, super sizing, and enormous
portions. Lightning fast technological advances providing "I want it now"
results have bled over into our health and wellness pursuit as well. To
avoid excess, a golden rule to follow is to eat when you're hungry and put
down your fork when you're full.

Excess Salt. We need salt to survive and for our bodies to function
properly. However, too much of a good thing is simply not good. Too
much salt will stop up your body's natural fluid flow. The body can hold
up to an average of 5 to 7 pounds of fluid after a good old Chinese meal.
Therefore, we need to become aware of our salt intake. Eliminate some
from your diet and you will soon find you are shedding excess fluid.
Drinking extra water will help to eliminate excess fluid, too.

Excess Sugars. An abundance of cookies, cakes, pies, and ice cream
will simply set you back weeks. Sometimes just eliminating these fun
foods for a while can kick start weight loss up to as much as 10 pounds
rather quickly, especially if you like them as much as I do.

If you find yourself living in excess, don't let this take you off course
in defeat. Start with small cutbacks. Great freedom is found in the small
choices. Don't give up on your day just because you made one, two, or
even three mistakes. I challenge you to fight excess moderately.

Do You Exercise Year-round?
Day 322

rest
day

Twenty percent of adult Americans work out year-round. This leaves eighty percent of adult Americans NOT working out year-round.

The recommended activity for adults is to get at least 2.5 hours of moderate intensity aerobic exercise each week. It's also recommended that adults should engage in muscle-strengthening activities like lifting weights or doing push-ups at least twice per week. These guidelines are very doable.

I think the biggest fascination that keeps the year-round exerciser exercising is the way it makes you feel. Once you experience the great feelings and benefits of exercise, it no longer feels chore-like; I like to call this the crossover. You've crossed over from the eighty percent to the twenty percent that exercises year-round. You're hooked on the feeling of exercise and can actually crave a workout, finding yourself irritable if you've missed one.

Less than 5% of adults participate in 30 minutes of physical activity each day; only one in three adults engage in the recommended amount of physical activity each week.

Only 35 – 44% of adults 75 years or older are physically active. You may be thinking, "what does it matter for the elderly?" It matters a lot. Exercise helps maintain bone density.

Children now spend more than seven and a half hours each day in front of a screen like the TV, video games, computer, etc.

Nearly one-third of high school students play video or computer games for 3 or more hours on an average SCHOOL day.

My hope and prayer is that the eighty percent group of Americans experience the crossover to year-round exercise. Major change is made in a culture one person at a time. I believe we can change these percentages in America and be a FIT, healthy, thriving nation.

In Search of Comfort
Day 323

I'm sure you have certain foods you gravitate toward that bring comfort. Comfort foods can mean different things to each individual, because they trigger personal memories. One common thread people have with comfort foods is that it brings feelings of comfort on any particular occasion. There's nothing wrong with this kind of eating until it interferes with your health.

Sometimes people run to certain foods to cope with life. When these foods are eaten repeatedly over a period of time, it can do damage to your wellness. I'll use myself as an example. Years ago, I would find comfort in eating a full bag of buttered popcorn. It brought a soothing feeling of when my momma used to make popcorn.

The only problem is that I didn't need the extra calories. These extra calories outweighed the comfort that bag of popcorn brought every night. It was always followed by mornings of misery, a puffy face, and a swollen body. I found I wasn't alone in this quest for false comfort. Others have told me similar stories of their comfort foods. Their eating habits left them feeling miserable, too.

In all circumstances, we may feel the need, out of habit, to search for a quick fix toward comfort food to help get us through the day. I guess the big question is, are the foods you're reaching for providing you with false comforts? I encourage you to take a look at your go-to habits. Are there any foods you need to let go of?

Be determined today to make the necessary changes. I assure you the real comfort you seek will be found.

Why Explosive Training?
Day 324

There are millions of ways to train. We should dabble in them all. I hope to encourage you to add some change to your normal routine. One way is by implementing "explosive training."

What is explosive training? It's high-intensity, short-duration resistance training, also known as burst training. This type of training produces results like nothing else. There are some good reasons why this type of training is like nothing else. Explosive training increases growth hormones and adrenaline release. This increase in growth hormones and adrenaline release is recognized as stress hormones in the body that stimulate fat breakdown.

Fat breakdown is the secret to reducing body fat. Explosive training triggers hormonal and central nervous system responses. It will help your body change from being a fat storer to a fat burner. It creates the correct hormonal balances that trigger hormone-sensitive lipase (which is an enzyme) that helps your body release fat from cells.

Here are some burst training exercises you can add to your workout. These particular exercises should not replace your routine but enhance your existing workouts. For instance, if you're doing bench presses, at the end of your set you can continue with bench presses and include high intensity, fast, short, explosive movements to end your set.

You can use a wide variety of exercises, but remember the key element here is working the large muscle groups with an overload stimulus: Barbell Bench Press, Bent-Over Rows, Barbell Squats, Shrugs Barbell Overhead Shoulder Press, Dead-Lifts.

Explosive training can also be done with bodyweight exercises. Commonly used in burst training: Push-ups, Pull-ups, Mountain Climbers, Bear Crawls, Leg Lifts, Plyo box jumps.

There are endless ways you can put together a burst training workout. Fitness is so fun. I challenge you to try it.

Muscles Must be Fed the Right Fuel
Day 325

If we're going to make the effort to exercise, of course we want results!! Have you ever felt like you're pedaling backwards instead of forwards in your health and wellness? The good news is that there may be an easy solution: Protein!

We need a constant reminder in a carbohydrate-crazed world. Don't forget protein! Our muscles must be fed the right fuel to respond. If you want to build muscle or lose weight, there's nothing more important you can add to your diet than protein.

Protein is an important factor in developing pretty muscles for the ladies and handsome muscles for the gentlemen. How much protein does the average person need? 20 grams are recommended for ladies and around 30 grams recommended for gentlemen at every meal.

The reason for this amount is because our bodies can only metabolize 20 to 30 grams at one sitting. Eating smaller portions more frequently throughout the day produces the best results. With smaller portions, your body is able to absorb the protein it needs to feed your muscles properly.

If you eat more protein than your body can metabolize at one meal, your body won't be able to process those extra calories, and they'll ultimately end up stored as fat.

Will cutting carbs help my muscles grow faster? Short answer: No. As effective as high-protein diets are for losing weight, you still need carbs and fat for maximum muscle growth. Your body uses carbs for energy while you exercise. If you don't get enough carbs in your daily intake, your body will use protein as an alternate fuel source. Keep your appetite in check.

Stay moderate and aware of your fuel sources. Take time to fuel up on the right blend. We train hard; let's feed our muscles to prove it.

How Super is Your Food?
Day 326

Eating vegetables may be the last thing on your mind, but make sure they are the first thing on your plate. But why choose just any vegetable when you can choose super vegetables?

While a wide variety of colorful fruits and vegetables are always recommended, there are a few that you may want to choose over others for their exceptional health benefits. Here are a few for your consideration:

Red – Pink grapefruit, red bell peppers, tomatoes, and watermelon. These show promise in fighting lung and prostate cancer.

Purple – Concord grapes, blueberries, and prunes. These may help ward off heart disease.

Green – Spinach, broccoli, Brussels sprouts, collard greens, and bok choy. Dark green leafy vegetables are usually high in vitamin B, which is another heart disease fighter.

Orange – Carrots, mango, pumpkin, and oranges. These help to reduce the risk of heart disease and improve immune function.

White – Cauliflower, mushrooms, banana, and onions. These help to lower blood pressure and may protect against stomach cancer.

Eat vegetables raw to get the greatest nutritional benefit. If raw is not an option, then choose the frozen version; if that isn't possible then choose the canned versions. I can tell you from experience that these vegetables will make your body feel super and function at its most efficient level.

We're supposed to have 7 servings a day. Let me encourage you to branch out and try a few new super fruits and veggies. Do your own research and see how you feel. I bet you will quickly find that you feel super.

Setting Our Sails Forward
Day 327

I'm going to share as if you have the same thought process of dreading the unknown. I'm one who resists the unknown because it's beyond my control. Funny? Sure, that's funny because we really don't ever have control of our future like we may think we do.

During the past 17 months, the new work style and new way of living has become the "new norm" for all of us. I've been calling it a "new norm" in hopes that we all can get back to what we call our personal "normal" soon. Well, soon has come and gone, so it's time for us to think of a new way to live our lives in a more healthy "thinking" kind of way.

I've made up my mind to no longer long for work as it was seventeen months ago, but to do my best today, looking toward the future. I'm going to look bright into today and for what tomorrow holds to create a better atmosphere for myself. Sure, this "new norm" has been extremely uncomfortable at times. I miss what once was, but I know now, no one knows what the future holds. We're all learning together.

I'm not going to look back on something that may never come back as it once was. The time is NOW … by golly, as we go forward let us make the choice to flip our thinking from negative to positive and embrace these days as normal.

I challenge you to handle whatever comes your way. Be determined to set your sails forward, forgetting about what lies behind once and for all. GOD'S GOT THIS. He holds the future in His hands.

Celebrate Mobility
Day 328

rest day

When I count my blessings, I always count the blessing of mobility twice! While I am thankful for the mobility provided by planes, trains, and automobiles, I am twice as thankful for the mobility provided by my body. What a great time of year to "exercise" this blessing.

As we celebrate the holidays with our family and friends and give thanks for our blessings, let's not forget to include the blessing of mobility. Oftentimes, during all the busyness brought on at this time of year, exercise goes to the wayside. This year, let's include a little exercise in our Thanksgiving season.

If you're in charge of the upcoming festivities, get creative and play yard games with the kids or orchestrate a walk with everyone. Any activity is good and goes a long way. Let's not take for granted the blessing to move our body.

Remember, movement is a gift. Fit it into your busy schedule. The choices we make today must be grounded in God's mercy and grace that is fresh and new every morning and not in yesterday's failures or victories or future fears.

I challenge you to celebrate your mobility.

Living a Healthy Lifestyle Together
Day 329

rest day My Pastor has always said, "You never know what a person is really made of until you see them walk through a trial!!" When someone is squeezed under pressure, what's really in a person's heart will come out.

Over the years, I've come to know a lot of beautiful people. While you may be beautiful on the outside, your true beauty is displayed when you're squeezed by the most tragic events or by the nagging stresses of work.

During this year, I'm sure you've walked through the most mundane days and the most eventful days as you've strived for better health. Living a healthy life isn't for the weak of heart. It takes commitment and loyalty to walk through the ups and downs of the pressures of life.

I believe health and wellness is a very personal thing. I take it very seriously to be a part of your life. Striving for better health is HARD and seems to be a trial all by itself. We all have our good and bad days and simply need the camaraderie and accountability to keep on track. Have you ever heard the saying, "It takes a village to raise a child?" It also takes a committed group of people to birth lasting fitness success. I always say that this journey is full of mountaintops and low valleys. There is something special about doing fitness together.

I'm so thankful you choose to walk out the most mundane to the most eventful days of life together. I wanted to say THANK YOU from the bottom of my heart for allowing me to live a healthy life together with YOU. I'm thankful you chose to do fitness with me this year. I pray I leave you with an undying love of fitness.

HAPPY THANKSGIVING!

Overcome by the Power of Your Testimony
Day 330

Do you know what happens when you talk about all the good that's happening in your life? Victory which produces more victories. By sharing the awesome things that are happening to you as a result of making exercise a regular part of your week, you're fanning the flame of hope in yourself and others.

In sharing your victories, you are defeating the negative voices that tell you otherwise. Revelation 12:11 is a scripture I love about overcoming through your testimony. It's worth reading so I hope you will look it up.

Here are some examples of the power of personal testimony.

A friend of mine started doing my daily workout videos. She had always jogged for her exercise but had never done any kind of resistance training. She made a new commitment to resistance training, and her husband noticed the tremendous difference in her body composition. Her body was firmer, more toned in her legs, glutes, upper body, and arms. She's tickled her husband noticed, and she's still onboard, motivated, and making incredible progress.

Another testimony is from a client who found her sweet spot by learning what regimen worked best for her body. She became extremely dedicated to rising early to train regularly, to eating well, and to dabbling in different types of fitness. Her testimony is one that confirms you can look your best if you continue to do what you know is right.

Don't overlook the power of a testimony. What you may think is seemingly insignificant is the very testimony that may be pushing you and others to overcome. We need a small army surrounding us who will share success stories to help each other achieve our best. You WILL overcome by the power of your testimony.

Guiltless You Time
Day 331

There's such a bad rap when it comes to setting aside some time just for yourself. Many people have the mistaken idea that in order to be successful in life, one must sacrifice everything, including "personal enjoyment."

When all you've ever done is give to others, leaving yourself depleted, you need to incorporate self care. When you're consumed with guilt and would never consider making the time, stop. Because everything else that you're striving for will suffer. I'm not suggesting excessive "you time," but moderately allow yourself the privilege to relax and regroup.

Let's create some "you time" with a few basic necessities of life. A great one is to go to bed around the same time every night. Have you ever felt guilty for sleeping? Do you think there's too much going on to get a good night's sleep? Rethink. Sleeping sets you up to better handle problems that arise daily. Give yourself permission to sleep.

Exercise guilt-free. Take time to find an exercise that works for you. Now-a-days, exercise has become so specialized that there's a "You Time" blessing to be discovered. The very first step is to seek enjoyment. Do your personal research and GO FOR IT…guilt-free. You must remember life is a gift.

We all get so busy. We feel as though we don't have time for this or that. But the truth of the matter is we can't afford NOT to make time to add some simple, guiltless "you time."

Sure, life has its ups and downs. So whatever each new day brings, it's much easier to digest when you feel better and healthier. I challenge you to utilize the basic necessities of life to your advantage. There are never any regrets when you're doing healthy things for yourself. It's always worth it.

I Want a Runner's High
Day 332

 A client of mine asked me about the "runner's high." She said she's never gotten that "feel-good" feeling from exercise that she's heard people mention.

What exactly is a runner's high and how can we experience it? The medical definition of a runner's high is "a feeling of euphoria that is experienced by some individuals engaged in strenuous running and that is held to be associated with the release of endorphins by the brain."

To produce endorphins, you have to push yourself hard enough to cause your body physical discomfort so it will release these painkiller chemicals. Usually Type A personality people seek after the runner's high. When you experience the release of these particular endorphins, you always want it again, and want more of it. Have you ever heard of an "endorphin junkie?" That explains the hardcore exerciser who is pursuing that runner's high. We must remember that if you fall under the category of an "endorphin junkie," your workouts should NOT be excruciating every time.

It's better to be on a quest to find a sweet spot where your workouts are comfortably challenging, so you can stay injury-free. For the more laid back personality who thinks endorphin junkies are crazy, your workouts are just as beneficial. When your heart rate is elevated, even training at a moderate pace, the serotonin chemical is being produced. You can still reach every single goal you'd like to accomplish.

Exercise is good. It produces feel-good chemicals. Even though the runner's high isn't for everyone, both the intense "endorphin junkie" and the laid back "serotonin producer" still reap benefits. Let's continue moving forward, joining arms with other like-minded people. There are different methods for achieving shared health and wellness visions and goals. Cheers to "getting high" the healthy way.

Peace of Mind
Day 333

Peace of mind is one of the greatest things in life to achieve. Our peace of mind is often threatened by life events which are out of our control. The 2020 Pandemic, for instance, affected us all. So what can bring you peace of mind? If you asked me that question, I would say reading the Bible every morning brings me the greatest peace of mind.

Second to that is exercise. It's true; effective exercise can positively affect your state of mind. When you exercise, your brain literally creates a mood-boosting chemical called serotonin. You signal your brain to increase serotonin production by working up a sweat.

People who are prone to depression often have low levels of serotonin. This partially explains why exercise can lower the risk of depression. For when your serotonin level is low, you don't often feel like getting off the couch to exercise. However, if you can stir-up enough self-encouragement to exercise, your energy level and spirits are guaranteed to be lifted.

Another brain chemical that helps with motivation and reward is dopamine. If you feel motivated and ready to tackle the day's list of projects after a workout, you can thank dopamine. It's what gives you the motivation to achieve something of value. Without enough dopamine, you probably wouldn't feel like putting forth the effort to do what you need to do. The fact exercise boosts the release of dopamine and serotonin can partially explain why exercise is a natural mood-lifting antidepressant.

I challenge you to look at exercise as something you can't wait to do. This will create the mental energy you need to keep going. For when you pursue peace of mind through exercise, you reap its benefits every single workout.

Are Pre-Packaged Low-Calorie Meals Healthy?
Day 334

When people make the decision to lose weight and strive for better health, the majority set out toward the freezer section and stock up on prepackaged meals, such as Lean Cuisines, Healthy Choice, Amy's Meals, etc. Most people think this is the better way.

These meals most definitely offer portion control, along with the meat and vegetable combination we need. But in some cases, these meals might NOT be the wisest choice to kick start weight loss or better heath.

These prepackaged foods have a lot of sodium. Too much salt results in water retention which makes weight loss difficult. The body has a harder time eliminating excess water and toxins from the body. High levels of sodium also cause inflammation in the joints of the body, which can cause pain.

Pre-packaged meals could hinder future success. If you never learn how to properly eat and rely on pre-packaged foods, it's hard to stick to a healthy diet in a non-pre-packaged world. Pre-packaged diet programs' success is short lived. The dieter doesn't know how to eat in a way that will sustain weight loss. Dieters seeking proper ways of losing weight keep the weight off longer than people who eat pre-packaged diet foods.

Pre-packaged meals are money makers. Participants that generally pay for their prepackaged meals in a weight loss program do have a major incentive to stick with their plan, but it's always short-term success.

I encourage all who desire a healthy future to learn all you can about the facts of food. Be leery if things seem too good to be true or too easy to do. They probably are. We're in this for the lifetime benefits of long-term good health.

Be Party Practical
Day 335

How many parties do have scheduled this month? Regardless of whether it's one or 21, you should plan on enjoying yourself while you're there. This is not the time to say, "Wow, I hope they have a lot of fresh celery available to eat, because that's all I want." While celery is a delicious little snack, I would encourage you to spread your wings and try a few other foods. Being party practical is the secret.

Party practical means it's okay for you to enjoy the different foods made available to you by simply using portion control. Portion control is being party practical at its best. December is a month to celebrate. I'm sure there are a lot of different things that we can eat that are only offered at this time of the year. Plan to partake in all you desire with portion control in mind.

The primary key in practicing successful portion control is to not show up to the party hungry. You want to make sure you aren't starving so you don't find yourself doing out-of-control grazing all night. A light healthy snack and some water can help fill the gaps before you get to the party.

This is a great time of year to be with family and friends. Enjoy them and enjoy the bounty of foods placed before you. Tis the season.

Holiday Food for Thought
Day 336

rest day Did you know that the average American gains one to two pounds during the holidays? That might not seem like much, but this small weight gain tends to stick and accumulate over the years. For example, if you're 30 years old and fall into allowing one to two pounds to stay from the holidays, by the age of forty you're 10 pounds heavier.

I have good news. Those pounds can be avoided by simply being mindful of what you're eating. Have you ever been cooking holiday candy or baked goods, and before you know it, you're stuffed and you're not even aware of what you've eaten? Or you're waiting for an evening holiday event, so you skip breakfast and lunch to prepare your tummy for all those special treats, only to find yourself stuffed from having eaten more than you should have?

There are ways around all the holiday fun without putting on any extra pounds.

Don't skip meals. In preparation for a big holiday party or evening event, contrary to thinking that skipping meals throughout the day is best…DON'T. It's about 75% guaranteed that your evening will end with overeating or over-drinking.

Moderation is key. We've heard this truth a bunch, right? Of course, holiday meals tend to be large, buffet style meals, encouraging second and third helpings.

There are many strategies to help you avoid overeating. Here are a couple of suggestions. Using a smaller plate, for instance, allows you to put less food on your plate and encourages proper portion sizes.

Welcome the distractions. Instead of going for a second food helping, get moving as a family. Being active is a great time to catch up with family members. Come up with your own family fitness traditions.

I challenge you to be mindful.

A Season to Enjoy
Day 337

My prayer for all my beautiful clients is to enjoy this season. I know, it's very hectic this time of year, let's not let it be a joy-killer. Life is supposed to be enjoyed. How can we do that? Eat and drink. The Bible even says so. Ecclesiastes 2:22-24 (NKJV) says,

"For what has a man for all his labor and for the striving of his heart with which he has toiled under the sun? Work is burdensome and at night the heart can take no rest. Is all vanity? So, there is nothing better for a man than he should eat and drink and that his soul should enjoy good in his labor."

I constantly have to remind myself to enjoy life. It may not have gone the way I'd like for it to go, but I'm determined not to be all grumpy about it and to find enjoyment in all the craziness life brings.

I'd like to share some simple mood lifters to keep you aboard the healthy train this holiday season week.

Don't allow your blood sugar to drop by forgetting to eat. Hunger can negatively affect your mood.

Make sure you're eating enough protein. Having the sufficient amount will help you feel alert and productive for hours.

Sleep is important. So don't let all the extra late night events cut into your sleep time. Most adults require between 7 and 9 hours of sleep per night, you might need slightly more or less to function optimally. The important thing is you consistently get the sleep you need.

I challenge you to engage in some kind of movement. If your normal session at the gym isn't an option, just get up and simply move to boost your mood and energy level.

Enjoy the season!

December Fitness is a Head Start
Day 338

You have daily decisions to make, and all your decisions have consequences, whether they're good or bad, big or small. I'd like to encourage you during this December month, when food options are plenty and the parties are roaring, to keep on the fitness path. The measly little choice to exercise makes a tremendous difference. Instead of being so food focused, I say, ENJOY and get a head start on the new year by keeping exercise a part of your December.

There are some simple ways to continue on your health path even during this holiday that can reap year round benefits. For instance, I ran into one of my precious clients the other day and she was excited to share that she and a co-worker had a walk and talk business meeting.

Here are some facts. If you walked for 10 minutes every workday at a moderate 3 mph pace, you'd burn about 1,000 calories a month and lose 3 pounds a year. When your cell phone rings, slip on your walking shoes and stroll the halls at work or take it outside. Workplaces now have the option of a standing desk. The average person burns 100 calories per hour sitting versus 140 per hour standing. Get on your feet two hours a day while you work, and you could drop an extra six pounds over the year.

Every small decision to keep your body moving matters. It's a head start into this new year because you love exercise, even in the month of December.

If Only...
Day 339

If Only...Let me begin by saying that nothing is impossible. The past is gone and we can't change one iota of it. However, the coming year is a whole other story just waiting for possibilities.

Be encouraged by a story of an amazing woman who is 60 years young:

"I am an educated and intelligent person; I am loving and kind; I am compassionate and giving; I am a Child of God, wife, mother, daughter, sister, and friend, but it frequently appeared to me that no one saw that in me because they couldn't get beyond the fat. I decided I was not going to live the rest of my life that way.

I prayed I would have the willpower and stamina to discover the body God gave to glorify Him. In August my employer made You Can Do Fitness classes available to my department. I jumped at the chance.

I could not even bend over and tie my own shoes when we started! I wanted to be able to tie my own shoes, fit into a booth at any restaurant, and to be able to fly without asking for a seat extension.

I also joined a national weight loss eating program. I learned new ways to count fat and calories and substitute foods and ingredients that made a lifestyle change possible for me.

Now I eat very different and have made exercise a crucial part of my life. I have lost almost 140 pounds. I have gone from a size 28 to a size 14 and I'm not done yet. I thank God for the fitness classes and finding a new way to eat."

I challenge you to turn your impossibilities to possibilities. Embrace the coming year. Seek new ways to become the next success testimony.

Be Exercise Practical
Day 340

Okay, so let's be real. With all the shopping, parties, and year-end work projects, our health and wellness routines often get pushed to the back burner. It becomes difficult to squeeze a workout in with all the demands of getting ready for the holidays.

Some kind of exercise is better than no exercise. So I suggest you find short periods of time to fit exercise into your day. Within that short time frame, I encourage you to work towards being what I call "exercise practical."

You are exercise practical when you take a high-priority event and figure out ways to fit exercise into it. For instance, you can get the family all bundled up in warm attire after dinner and take a walk through the neighborhood to see the Christmas lights. You can also use Christmas shopping as an opportunity to get in a little cardio exercise by walking from one end of the mall to the other instead of getting in your car and driving around the mall to get there. As your trainer, I wouldn't insist you do walking lunges as you walk to the other side, but you could. Just imagine the looks you would get! If you don't care what people think, you should definitely do the walking lunges. You can add bicep curls while holding heavy shopping bags for a bigger challenge.

These suggestions come honestly; I've done them all. Stay determined to keep up the good work because all movement matters. Know that when the new year is here, you'll be on track and the challenges in your new workout routine will be much easier because you've been exercise practical.

Have No Doubt ... It's Working
Day 341

My daughter got the fitness bug in her early teens. Patience was a recurring theme when answering her 101 questions. Kids are generally more impatient than adults, but when it comes to fitness results, children and adults are alike. When you work hard, you want to see results and see them now.

It's important to know that what you're doing is working. Here are some questions my daughter asked:

How long after you start working out do you gain muscle? There are a lot of variables that play into how quickly you gain muscle or strength after you start working out diligently. Baseline fitness, genetics, diet, specific training methods, gender, and age all play into how quickly you can gain muscle and strength. Generally speaking, men can add between 1.5 – 2.5 pounds of muscle every month. Women put on muscle mass at a slower rate than men (largely due to testosterone levels), roughly half as fast as men or about ½ pound every 2 weeks, or 1 pound per month.

How soon will I start losing weight? When you implement a regular exercise regime, you can see a difference in the numbers on the scale in as little as a week. If you combine your physical activity with healthy eating changes and reasonable calorie consumption, you can easily drop 2 pounds per week.

How long after working out until I start to look more toned? When you train on a regular basis, you can see a difference in the form of more muscle definition in as little as two weeks. A focus on strength training makes the body feel "hard" and gives it the appearance of being more defined.

Be encouraged!! Have no doubt. It's working!! Time and commitment will get you the results you want to see.

Learning Your Body Daily
Day 342

rest day If you play a sport, or have some kind of physical disability, you know about body assessment. An athlete does a body assessment prior to a particular athletic event. It's just as important for you to assess your body daily to see if you're feeling okay before you begin your day.

Pregnant women often learn to assess their body all throughout their pregnancy. It's significant to take inventory of your body. The longer you're on this ol' earth, the more you need to learn about your own body's aches and pains.

I'd like to share a recent experience with you; I was having some lower back pain. I had pretty severe pain after my five-day workout week. I listened to the pain and took extra caution. Going into the weekend, I rested more than I usually would've, so I could start my work week rested and ready to go. Monday came around and I was still pretty tight, but knowing I had just rested two days before, I knew it was time to push through with some movement. By the end of that work week, I finally felt a release.

The moral to the story is, I had to assess my body's needs daily, whether that be to rest or move. It takes some learning to know exactly what your body needs. I believe oftentimes we either move too early in the healing process, or we get too much rest and we're sore from resting longer than our body needs.

Your body changes. It's your job to learn all the new ways of caring for yourself. Embrace inevitable change. Some body changes produce challenges. But with joy and thanksgiving, I challenge you to continue to keep active. Exercise is the best gift you can give yourself.

V-I-C-T-O-R-Y
Day 343

rest day Did you exercise today? Victory! Did you walk an extra 10 minutes today? Victory! Did you say yes to a healthy snack? Victory! Did you push away from the table? Victory!

Victory is a rewarding consequence of your plan being put into action. It's the everyday choices you make that are the very stepping and shaping stones of who you are today. You must pause during your day and seek out the good you've done. What you don't recognize won't stay. So, recognize the choices you've made toward a healthier lifestyle.

If you've found yourself walking in a stream of decisions that haven't been good lately, don't stop there. What you recognize, you can change. Now you recognize what you can be doing better — make a change, keep moving. It matters!

Plan now not to eat that extra cookie, brownie, etc., and then when the temptation arises, put that plan into action. Every choice makes a difference. A plan without action will render nothing. A plan with action will bring about victory. Then one day you'll look back and go, "Wow, I'm walking in victory."

It's the very choices you're making today that are shooting you straight into your victory land.

A victorious life of fitness is within your power. Recognize your good and bad. Grab your day by the horns and make your victory happen.

Steamroller Determination
Day 344

Steamroller determination. That's the first description that came to my mind when I thought about my client's success. Have you ever seen a steamroller in action? When there is a task or an obstacle set before the machine to conquer, it will overcome it, regardless.

Life is unpredictable and full of unforeseen matters, including health issues that seem to come out of nowhere. That's what my client faced last year. But her steamroller determination kept her pursuing a life of fitness:

"There have been many things going on with me this year health wise, and through all of it I have kept encouraged and motivated. I have not given up, and even though I might not have been able to do everything every week, I kept pushing myself. I know I have only lost 5 pounds this year, but that's okay because I have strengthened myself and I know the weight will come off."

I applaud my client for her strength and her drive. Regardless of her obstacles, she has found a way to continue her pursuit of fitness, health, and wellness. Her determination to remain active and mobile gives her the courage to get back up every time she is knocked down.

So when life knocks you in the nose, don't let it stop you. Get back up. In this ol' world you're bound to get hit more than once. It's how we respond to the trouble at hand. I challenge you not to react but instead use a steamroller determination. Use fitness to cope with obstacles while you keep pursuing a life of fitness, health, and wellness. You'll come out healthier.

Specific Stretching
Day 345

Stretching in general is always good. Today I'd like to share a certain type of stretching that may help and work for you. This particular type of stretch is called Active Isolated Stretching (AIS). I like to say it's a stretch with purpose. You isolate the muscle to be stretched by actively contracting the opposite muscle.

For Example: If you are aiming to stretch the hamstrings (the muscles on the back of the thigh), you must first actively contract the quadriceps (the muscles on the front of the thigh). Then, the brain sends a signal to the hamstrings to relax. This provides a perfect environment for the hamstrings to stretch. Repeating each stretch eight to 10 times increases the circulation of blood, oxygen, and nutrients to the muscles being stretched.

This technique will help an individual gain the most flexibility per session. The more nutrition a muscle can obtain and the more toxins a muscle can release, the faster the muscle can recover. The reason for such a short hold is because it avoids the activation of the stretch reflex. This stretch reflex is like a safety mechanism that activates it to prevent a muscle or tendon from overstretching too far or too fast.

In all my years of schooling, I've been taught to advocate that stretching should last up to 60 seconds. This prolonged static stretching technique was the gold standard. Prolonged static stretching can actually decrease the blood flow. With a decrease in blood flow, the muscle tissue is creating the very thing we are trying to get rid of, which is lactic acid buildup. This can potentially cause irritation or injury to the muscles.

You can do the standard 60-second hold stretching after your exercise session. You can do a little AIS, too. Both have benefits.

Goodness Follows Exercise
Day 346

Who in the world doesn't want goodness in their lives? Everyone wants goodness in their lives. When you think of goodness, what comes to mind? I'll bet we can share desired goodness.

Good Health: Who doesn't desire good health...? Without GOOD health we can't enjoy what we love doing most. I've heard many times in my industry, "Health is your first wealth." If you could have everything money could buy, but weren't in good health, you couldn't enjoy it.

Exercise brings a plethora of goodness. If I could interview you, I imagine you'd tell me many good things that happened to your health when you made exercise a priority.

Good Company: Who is in your immediate circle of friends? Believe it or not, it matters. We're extremely influenced by who we hang around. Having the honor of being in the fitness industry, I've not only gotten the privilege to help others, but had the opportunity to be around individuals that want to better themselves. This has pushed me to continue to grow. I've been challenged, prodded, and encouraged. I continue to learn so much by being in the company of amazing people.

Results: The beauty of exercise is that goodness ALWAYS comes in the form of results. The key is to always be looking for any good that may come. It may not come exactly like you thought it would, but if you're a goodness seeker you'll find the good. If you're a fault seeker you'll find fault. Remember, you ALWAYS find what you seek.

To conclude, we are all after good health. Your motivation may be to lower blood pressure, prevent diabetes, look your best on your wedding day, prepare for surgery, or many more scenarios. Nevertheless, the goal of achieving something good is the same. Goodness follows exercise.

Krebs Cycle
Day 347

I'd like to touch on the Krebs Cycle. I'm no biochemical scientist, but I would like take this biochemical term and simplify it to better understand this particular energy pathway we all want to reach. How do I know you want to reach this energy pathway? Because within "The Krebs Cycle" is where your carbohydrate/fat conversion is utilized.

The Merriam-Webster definition of Krebs Cycle is "a sequence of re-actions in the living organism in which oxidation of acetic acid or acetyl equivalent provides energy for storage in phosphate bonds (as in ATP) — called also citric acid cycle, tricarboxylic acid cycle."

If that sounds like a bunch of Mumbo Jumbo to you, it does to me, too. But it's so very important for us to understand the basics of the Krebs Cycle.

When we exercise, our bodies utilize three main metabolic path-ways:

- ATP-CP - This first pathway is utilized when you exert yourself with a quick burst of maximum energy of a minute or less.

- Then your body goes into utilizing your second energy pathway, known as the glycolytic pathway. It's very short, lasting 1-3 minutes. These first two pathways use zero oxygen.

- Then the 3rd energy pathway requires oxygen. Any exercise re-quiring oxygen brings us to the Krebs Cycle. When oxygen is required, it's to help you to continue performing the task.

To simply put this without getting over my own head, the Krebs cy-cle is the only way that FAT gets used in energy production. The more TIME that you exercise, the more that ENERGY is used. The body then switches from burning more carbohydrates to burning more fat for ener-gy. This takes place around sixteen minutes.

Again, sixteen minutes is the carbohydrate/fat conversion. Who knew sixteen minutes could be so magical?

Why Your Workouts May Not Be Effective
Day 348

It's a no-brainer how fantastic working out is for your health. But what happens when your workouts aren't delivering the results you want? While any kind of physical activity is good, some workout plans are better than others. A lot of factors come into play when trying to lose weight and tone up.

If your workout isn't working for you, you may consider some reasons why:

You may not be working out hard enough. If you've been exercising consistently for several weeks, months, or years, it's definitely time to increase the intensity and start pushing yourself. You can begin regularly pushing yourself beyond your fitness comfort zone. Whether you increase the frequency, intensity, or duration of your workouts, you have to switch it up.

You might be rewarding yourself with food unaware. You'll be hungrier and need to monitor your intake. You might allow yourself to have that extra piece of pizza or order dessert because you "went to the gym" earlier. I'm guilty. If so, you may be undoing all of that good calorie burning with too many treats.

You may sit all day. Sure, you work out regularly, but what you do the rest of the day matters, too! If you put in a solid exercise session only to sit at a desk all day, you may be plateauing all of your hard work at the gym. Try adding more activity during your work day. You could even set a timer to beep every half hour to remind you to stand up, stretch, and do a quick lap around the office/parking lot.

You must be methodical about your next move all the time, learning new ways to stay effective. The rewards are worth the investment. There is only one you, and you're worth it.

Be a Rebel!
Day 349

rest day Go against the grain this holiday season and keep exercising. People are notorious for dropping out of the gym this time of the year. They prefer to put all the pressure on themselves to start back up on January 1st.

From firsthand experience, I know it's easier to just keep going than to stop and hope to start back up on an appointed date. There is always a chance you won't start back up on January 1st. Then, you'll be left feeling defeated and depressed, and who knows when or if you'll get going again.

Be a rebel this time of year and don't let this happen to you. You mustn't follow the pack and take a big break. Tell your friends who may be considering an exercise break, "DON'T DO IT!"

Keep your fitness boat afloat and don't pull the plug. It's in times like these the little things make a big difference. Maintaining a consistent workout schedule will guarantee you do not undo what you've worked so hard to accomplish.

Trust me on this one. I've dropped the ball too many times during this month only to greet January depressed and with extra weight to lose. By keeping your fitness boat strong and steady, you'll end this year and begin the new year with a tremendous sense of accomplishment. Then in January, you can take your workout up to a new fitness level because you'll be ready for the challenge.

So keep going and stay strong. Be a rebel for a great cause. You're definitely worth it.

I'm So Bored I Could Scream!
Day 350

rest day   Even the most eager, dedicated fitness enthusiast gets bored with exercise. No one is immune to an exercise slump. One time or another, you'll be filled with a lack of inspiration, or low motivation. When this happens, dig deep and make a change before an exercise slump becomes a fitness derailment.

It's normal to get bored when you're looking at the same machines/fitness videos and are doing the same routine every single day. We all have a common link of wanting to stay motivated. We want to continue to see results and enjoy our fitness.

Here are some slumps and strategies for overcoming them:

Slump #1. Doing the same exercise for the same body part every workout. You must realize doing bicep curls, chest presses, triceps extensions, or squats the same way every workout will set you up for injury, a fitness plateau, or plain old boredom.

Strategy? If you train chest 3 days a week, you need to change up the type of chest exercises you're doing. For instance, do flat bench dumbbells on Monday. Wednesday, do cables crossovers. Friday, do straight bar bench presses.

Slump #2. Doing your workouts in the same order. Boring.

Strategy? Change your order. Do strength training before cardio or vice versa. Changing the order by tweaking your routine will produce strength gains. This will put some excitement back into your workouts.

Slump #3. Neglecting your existing exercise routine. Your routine needs constant attention.

Strategy? Change your focus. When first starting any exercise program, a 3-day total body workout is best. As you get stronger, it's time to up your intensity. It's a must to keep yourself challenged.

It's guaranteed you'll be bored with workouts. Simply be prepared. Remember, feeling bored doesn't mean it's quitting time. Boredom is just a signal for change.

New
Day 351

When I say the word "new," I'll bet good things come to mind. Maybe you're thinking about a new car, new home, new baby, new marriage, new date, new job…and the list goes on. I always wake up early to have my cup of joe with Jesus, and this morning, that word, "new," resonated deep within my soul. My life consists of the same schedule/routine day after day, year after year. I just completed homeschooling my two beautiful girls this year. My youngest just graduated from high school.

Talk about doing the same thing for many years in a row. My girls and I did the same thing together for 14 years. Talk about the word "new!" This year is a new one, alright. The Bible says in Lamentations 3:22-23, "It is because of the Lord's mercy and lovingkindness that we are not consumed, because His [tender] compassions fail not. They are NEW every morning; great and abundant is Your stability and faithfulness."

I'm 55+ years old. I've decided to replace my bad word "old" for "NEW" and tell myself this is a new day. I have new opportunities to make good choices. It's a must to become relentless in seeking out new things when new obstacles arise, until you find success.

I have a new daily determination to flip from thinking old or older into really pondering all the "NEW" and endless possibilities to doing something new. I hope and pray that you can get just as excited about the word "new," too. Because it's the truth.

Even on the mundane days of doing the same old thing, you get a new day to find your new. You have a new start to do the next right thing. See you on video for another new workout.

What is the Best Way to Lose Weight?
Day 352

I know the topic of weight loss is usually on the back burner of everyone's mind this time of year, but I wanted to plant a little seed with the new year right around the corner. I've had the honor of training a new client who has already lost over 85 pounds.

She shared her story of what it takes to lose weight the right way. There is no short cut. The formula is … determination and hard work!! None of us really want to hear this because as time goes by and technology advances, there will be no other way.

The best way to lose weight is to be dedicated for the long haul. Know up front there will be a lot of hard work involved. Implementing new things always requires change. We must remember that a lifestyle change requires time. Adapting to new ways, identifying current behaviors or habits that have led to weight increase, and replacing them with healthier habits takes time.

Behavior modifications do not take place overnight and are really tough to overcome sometimes, but it IS possible. It's a must to buckle up and accept the new you you're evolving into. Many times I've seen clients (including myself) not accept the good about themselves. We must embrace the good and positive changes that we've made and celebrate. If we don't, we run the risk of becoming discouraged, even depressed, and giving up.

Allow your fitness family or co-workers to point out all the results they see. Receive compliments! You've earned them! You're not going to get a big head; you need that encouragement.

I encourage you to believe you can do anything you set your mind to. With determination and hard work, your possibilities are endless. Because you can do fitness.

I've Blown It! What Now?
Day 353

 Have you ever eaten too much? Holiday parties, gourmet meals, and celebratory dinners can easily get more out of control than you expect. Let's face it; everyone blows his or her calorie budget every now and then. But I'm not here to talk about excessive calories today. I'm here to talk about the guilt and shame that follow a full belly.

That old dieter's saying, "a moment on the lips, forever on the hips" does NOT have to be true. Here are what medical experts, registered dietitians, and weight management specialists say about the damage done by one-time splurges.

Relax! The good news is one meal is NOT going to ruin you. Simply eat sensibly and exercise regularly the rest of the day or week. Remember, you need 3,500 calories to gain one pound of body fat.

Don't beat yourself up! Most people overeat somewhere between 500 and 1,500 calories every single day. There is an easy fix - eat consciously.

Forgive yourself. Dust off your feet. Don't stay there. Stop worrying. Choose to eat lighter during the week to make up for your fun time at the party … guilt free.

Skip the scale! After a feast, your weight is bound to be inflated. That's not because of an increase in body fat, but usually it's due to water retention brought on by the excess calories and salt you likely ate. Give your body a couple of days to regulate itself. Don't weigh yourself. Why put yourself though the extra stress of a higher number on the scale?

Refuse to allow defeat to be a part of your thought process. Be determined to press forward. You will make mistakes, BUT by golly, you won't camp there. The victory is in the rebound. Don't stop … get it … get it. :)

Steady to the End
Day 354

I'd like to give you some simple tips to stay steady until the end of the year. Facts never change. One big fact is a pound of fat is equivalent to 3,500 calories. In other words, at this time of year it's really easy for your caloric intake to exceed your caloric output, leaving you a pound or two heavier. BUT, if you increase your physical activity levels, you could keep yourself in balance throughout this fun time of year.

What does a pound or two matter in the big scheme of things, you might ask? Well, the truth is, pounds can add up quickly. The average person gains 7-10 pounds between Thanksgiving and the New Year. As simple as it is to gain weight, it's just as simple to keep it off. As your personal trainer, I'm challenging you to add just 10 little minutes of extra physical activity to the next two weeks. Not too sure what you can do?

Here are a few examples of exercises and the calories you can burn in just 10 minutes.

Walking at a brisk pace = 54 calories burned

Heavy cleaning = 54 calories burned

Using stairs = 175 calories burned

Raking leaves = 40 calories burned

I hope each and every one of you is blessed beyond measure. I pray you receive abundant benefits in your health and wellness from your faithful year with me.

Remember it doesn't take much. Just 10 minutes of physical activity goes a long, long way. Let's finish this year off right. Eat, drink, MOVE, and be merry.

Ho, Ho, Ho...'Tis the Season
Day 355

A year can bring a lot. Maybe it was a year of sudden change, isolation, sadness, or tragedy. These changes can leave you with a big choice: live in crippling fear or push forward in faith simply to survive. Maybe it was a year of bliss with abundant blessings: a new birth, a new marriage, or a new job. Happiness makes it much easier to move into a new year.

It's a must to use determination to rise up daily and immediately focus on what you have. You've got the certainty of change. Are you good with change? I'm not; it places me in a position to either choose to crawl under the table and curl up in a ball, full of anxiety, or to take the change on the chin and push forward. I encourage you to choose to push forward.

Looking back over this past year, my particular change has been the biggest blessing in disguise. I'm most thankful for my girls and my health. I'm also thankful for a social media platform to do my job. This change to social media has allowed me to keep my head in the game, have purpose to help others, and provide for my little family all at the same time.

I'll bet you have some things to reflect upon, too. If this has been a hard year, don't lose hope. Let's believe things will be better one day and a new, good norm will arise. Be determined to set your sails toward the future, welcoming the good ahead and leaving the bad behind.

I encourage you to cherish what you have this Christmas. Love one another every last step of this year. I love and appreciate YOU. Thank you for allowing me to be your personal trainer.

Fried Chicken -vs- Baked Chicken
Day 356

At the dinner table, when my kids were small, I often looked at their fried chicken then looked at my baked chicken, always amazed that eating fried chicken can have such different effects on the body than baked chicken. Whether it's fried chicken or anything that's full of empty calories, healthy choices must be a part of our weekly eating.

What are healthy choices? Eating lots of vegetables, lean meats, fruits, whole grains, and water. You may be rolling your eyes right now and telling yourself I know this stuff, but it's still the truth. Healthy habits, such as eating well, exercising, and avoiding harmful substances, are a no brainer but worth the reminder.

Every day people stop making healthy choices. Healthy habits are hard to develop and often require changing your mindset. But if you're willing to keep making healthy choices, the impact is powerful regardless of your age, sex, or physical ability.

Healthy reminders:

Controls weight. No matter what you weigh, if you're making healthy food choices you're controlling your weight.

Improves mood. Confidence arises after making good healthy food choice -vs- if you've eaten unhealthy, shame comes with it.

Boosts Energy. Food is a great acting agent for feeling like Popeye or a Debbie Downer. I encourage you to take note on how you feel after you've eaten a spinach salad -vs- how you feel after a McDonald's meal.

Nutrition Deficiency. "Empty calories" is the nutrient intake of high calorie foods that has little to no benefits for your health and negatively impacts your malnutrition.

The next time you have the opportunity to make a choice between fried or baked, choosing baked makes a difference. Don't ever grow weary in making good eating choices. Choose the baked chicken … you're worth the work.

Don't Be Stressed
Day 357

rest day Have you ever been so stressed that you know it's affecting your physical body? Then, when you're feeling the effects of stress, it makes you even more stressed?

Stress is a silent killer that must be reckoned with, or it can cause physical harm. But the hard part is, you just can't say, "don't be stressed;" stress doesn't magically go away. An outlet is needed to alleviate the physical trauma that stress causes to your physical body.

Finding an outlet to alleviate unwanted stress is important due to the number of health problems related to stress. Learning some basic stress relief techniques can go a long way.

Here are four stress-relief tips:

Exercise. Exercise is one of the best ways to manage stress. The number one reason this is true is because during exercise, chemicals are released by the body that counteract the negative substances secreted during a stressful situation.

Breathe deeply. Just a few minutes of deep breathing can help the physiologic stress response that is occurring when you are experiencing an unpleasant moment. One advantage to deep breathing for stress relief is that you can do it anywhere.

Focus on movement. Take a walk, and while you're walking, focus on the physical act of walking itself. Doing some kind of movement is a great way calm you down by bringing yourself back to the present moment. This may sound pretty cliché, but try it.

Life throws us curve balls that must be handled. When those hard knocks in life hit us, we might as well square our shoulders, hold our heads up high, and push forward in managing our stress the right way.

Intermittent Fasting
Day 358

Intermittent fasting (IF) is a way of eating which has proven to be successful for some individuals. IF is a plan where individuals consume any calorie-producing foods and beverages for just four to six hours a day for five days and consume a very low calorie diet the remaining days. The intermittent fasting days alternate with the "normal eating" days within the allotted schedule.

IF has proven to be an effective healing tool for a couple of reasons. For one, by giving our bodies a break from normal calorie consumption, our digestive tracts can actually heal. Secondly, people often find it to be an easy plan to follow even for those who don't like the hunger of dieting. It makes them feel better and quite often they lose weight.

Let's establish when IF is NOT for you. If you are pregnant or planning to become pregnant in the future of if you currently have or are recovering from an eating disorder, IF is NOT a healthy choice for you. Neither is IF a healthy choice if you are diabetic. Diabetes requires you to have a more equal distribution of food intake and to take certain medications that require specific food intake patterns.

I must say that I'm NOT a registered dietitian. So, I highly recommend that you make a quick call or visit to your doctor or Registered Dietitian Nutritionist (RDN) to get the green light before starting IF or any other new eating program.

Remember, no matter which eating style you choose, the goal is to stay mindful of your food choices for all meals and snacks. For when you manage your food intake wisely, you will feel better as you become a healthier and lighter version of you.

Dear Santa
Day 359

Merry Christmas, Fitness Friends!
I decided to have a little talk with Santa.

Dear Santa:

I know that you're getting ready for your big flight this week, but I just wanted to take a moment of your time to share my wish list with you. I have the greatest job in the world. I am a personal fitness trainer for a tremendous group of people. I have the honor of helping them achieve their health and wellness goals. Of all their goals, improved mobility and optimum health remain the ultimate gifts of all.

Only through their hard work and determination have they achieved these gifts of improved mobility and optimum health. If your elves are ever sneaking around, they will see my clients doing things that they never thought possible. While the flying reindeer thing you have going on still seems a little impossible to me, let me tell you that these people and their achievements are for real. They now take on what they once considered impossible physical feats and enjoy simple things, like walking the zoo with their children. They can now travel with their loved ones and hike Mount Everest or the Grand Canyon. Their commitment to fitness has exceeded their own expectations.

Well, Santa, I don't have a wish list, but I wanted to share what hard work and dedication can do. I am so blessed to have been given the opportunity to work with these people. My hope and prayer is each person that walked this fitness journey with me has a newfound love for working out.

I challenge everyone to have a great rest day. Calories don't count on holidays.

Merry Christmas to all, and to all a wonderful, healthy, and mobile life.

ALMOST A NEW YEAR
Day 360

 The last week of the year is what I like to call "forgotten week." It is tempting to put our health and wellness aside as we celebrate the new year. I find "forgotten week" to be a good time to set goals and wrap up fitness odds and ends like the ones below.

Set realistic goals. Make sure you set some reachable goals for yourself in the new year. Losing one or two pounds a week is doable. Remember we're in this for a lifetime. Slow weight loss equals keeping if off. Quick weight loss usually means you'll be more apt to gain it back.

Make weekly resolutions. Small goals develop into great victories. Over the years, I've seen people (myself included) who set their goal "really big" but don't have a small plan for achieving it. They end up getting frustrated and giving up. We must set weekly achievable goals and make one change at a time.

Celebrate your progress. When you achieve the first 10% of your long-range weight-loss goal, CELEBRATE! Recognizing your small victories will set you up for the best chance of ultimate success. Long-term weight loss is a slow but rewarding process.

Go easy on the alcohol. Remember that alcohol is a source of calories. Make sure to account for your alcohol calories by eliminating those extra food carbohydrates.

We sometimes forget that our bodies are ever-changing. We, therefore, need to frequently update our health and wellness goals and routines to address these changes. Our health is worth our utmost attention.

Renewal
Day 361

I hope you're filled with a renewal of hope, strength, inspiration, and most importantly, the peace of God, this season. There's a special bond that comes with exercising together. It creates a beautiful family tie. Through trials and victories this life is guaranteed to bring, we need a close-knit family to pull us up or pat us on the back during it all. The structured support of having each other is a constant need on this fitness journey.

Together we can keep the right focus in pointing each other toward physical blessings. So many of us struggle with distorted body image and feel grave disappointment in our journey. By keeping one another focused on blessings, it can bring renewal and draw us away from our imperfections. We must be reminded that every drop of sweat is a calorie burned, and we share that accomplishment together, come rain or shine.

Let's accept where we are and give ourselves the grace to continue to carry out this lifetime commitment of health and wellness. You've exercised consistently long enough to know that it's not the most popular or exciting task to do day in and day out. But, we have our faithful fitness friends to guide us.

I want to thank you for allowing me to be a part of this very special area of your life. I too receive a renewal of hope and strength from you. I'm inspired by every fitness victory shared from your hard work.

Why Warm Up or Cool Down?
Day 362

Here's why a warmup and cool down is vital. A warmup can be looked at like a fresh piece of gum. Gum straight from the wrapper isn't pliable. It can be broken very easily. Your body is the same way; at the beginning of a workout, it's stiff and at risk of being easily pulled, strained, or sprained. Fresh gum becomes pliable within a couple of chews just like your body, with a good warmup, becomes pliable, too.

The cool down is just as serious. I like to look at a cool down like ironing. After a good workout, your muscles are all pumped up, shortened and full of lactic acid, just like a wrinkled shirt needs to be ironed. A cool down needs its shortened muscles ironed out, assisting in homeostasis of an elevated heat rate and nice long muscles, too.

The warmup and cool down make or break a great workout. I'd like to share a sample warmup and cool down.

A warmup should begin with slow-paced aerobic activity, such as walking on a treadmill or easy pedaling on a stationary bicycle. Your warmup should take 5 to 10 minutes. You'll feel revived and ready for more of a challenge.

A cool down looks a lot like the warm up but comes right after your intense workout. As you're approaching the end of your exercise session, you'll begin to slow down your pace with more continuous low-impact movements. This continued movement is keeping your heart rate and blood pressure from dropping too rapidly, ironing out the blood supply that's mostly in your extremities to the normal blood flow process.

A warmup and cool down is essential for every single workout. I challenge you to take the time for both.

The Human Body Fuel Gauge
Day 363

rest day This morning on your way to work, I'll bet you checked your fuel gauge. It's also important to check your body's fuel gauge. Just as you stop for car fuel, you also need to stop and think about your food fuel.

Similar to thinking about what gas station you'll be stopping in for gas, you can think and plan what you will be eating to stay on track. Once you have a tentative food plan for the day, you will need to stay in tune to your hunger gauge, just like you would when your car gauge gets low.

A vehicle's fuel gauge tells you when to fill up and how much fuel your car needs. It's equally important to assess your hunger gauge. If you were to overfill your car tank, it would run out and get all over the ground. If you overfill your tummy tank, your excess has to be stored elsewhere. That "elsewhere" is usually stored in unwanted places.

Can you break your tummy fuel gauge? Yes, it can be broken by overeating meals and snacks. We can find ourselves in a rut, turning to food for comfort or to meet emotional needs. Food does NOT meet emotional needs or comfort.

How do you get your fuel gauge working again? It's really as simple as tremendously cutting back on the amount of food you consume. Allow your tummy to growl and experience hunger.

Remember to do a quick assessment. Be aware of every bite and check your fuel gauge during every meal. How much fuel do you need? Is your tummy on a 1/4 of a tank? 1/2 a tank? 3/4 full? We can't do without food, so we might as well learn all we can about our body.

Hungry?
Day 364

When you think of the word "hungry" do you associate it as a bad thing or a good thing? There's a lot of confusion when it comes to hunger. I've been asked really good questions from clients over the years. Examples: "Do you need to be hungry to lose weight? How do you know if you are truly hungry? How do I know if I'm just emotionally eating?"

You don't have to be hungry to lose weight. If you start to eat better, cut back on calories, or change things up, you might have to battle cravings or thoughts that you may be hungry.

You may turn to food for comfort, consciously or unconsciously. When facing difficult problems, feeling stressed, or even feeling bored, make sure you stay aware of how you're feeling and ask yourself lots of questions around food, like "Am I really hungry?" "What have I eaten so far today?" "Am I mad, sad, stressed, or depressed?" Be very careful to keep your emotions in check.

What is hunger? It's a compelling need or desire for food. You may experience it like a gnawing in the pit of your stomach. Your stomach may growl; you may feel lightheaded or even feel weak. When you experience these cues, your body is communicating a need for fuel.

Hunger is not to be feared. Being hungry makes me feel uncomfortable. I don't trust myself to make good decisions when I'm hungry. I have a safeguard plan of how much food I eat. I portion my food by eating out of measuring cups. I'm learning that hunger is not to be feared, but to be embraced and enjoyed.

Hunger is neither good or bad, wrong or right, it just is. I challenge you to learn your hunger cues.

Lean, Mean Muscle Machine
Day 365

The year can get away from us quickly, so encouragement is a necessity for keeping your body lean and muscular for the new month and new year ahead. Things you wouldn't think of as being motivating are the very things that keep us subconsciously motivated.

Things like:

Dressing for success: Wearing the appropriate clothing to get in the mindset of movement. As soon as the workout clothes go on, your mind should go right into exercise mode.

Do 20 jumping jacks. The hardest part of getting started in a workout is, well, getting started! So instead of setting a daunting goal of a 60-minute cardio session, start small. Promise yourself that you just have to do 5-10 minutes. Start off with something easy and manageable, such as 20 jumping jacks. Once you get going, you'll forget why it was so hard to get started in the first place.

Assessment check: Looking at yourself in the mirror. Mirrors don't lie, but it'll keep you honest with yourself. Please be kind to yourself as you take a peek at your body; don't be critical. Allow the mirror to be motivating with encouraging talk of positive thoughts and affirmations. With encouragement, improved body image comes by continuing to take good care of yourself. Instead of thinking, "I have big legs," change your thought to, "I have strong legs." Before you know it, your "problem areas" will no longer be your biggest enemy.

Reminding yourself why you sought out better health for yourself in the first place. Does diabetes run in your family? Are you unable to keep up with your kids? Do you want to feel more comfortable in a swimsuit? Don't forget why.

I challenge you to fight for your muscle machine.

Tell Me About Your Year

1. What are your sleep patterns?
   a) What time do you get up? _____
   b) What time do you go to bed? _____
   c) What time of day do you have the most energy? _____
   d) When is your favorite time of day to eat? _____

2. When is your biggest meal:
   _____ Breakfast
   _____ Lunch
   _____ Dinner

3. What type of foods are you drawn to?
   _____ Sweets (cake, candy, pies, etc)
   _____ Salts (chips, crackers, etc)
   _____ Fats (cream sauces, butter, etc)

4. What are you doing for exercise now? _____
   _____
   _____

5. Where do you exercise? _____
   a) How often do you exercise? _____
   b) When do you exercise? _____

6. If you could change one thing about your life what would it be?_____
   _____
   _____
   _____

I challenge you to stay aware of where you are in your fitness journey. Awareness is the only thing that will prompt us to change. We can't change what we're not aware of.

Contact me by email jadekrauss@gmail.com

About the Author

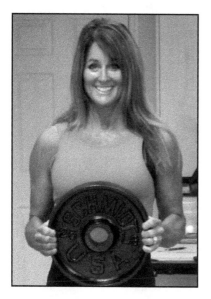

Jade (Krauss) Thornton was born in East Tennessee then headed to Tampa, FL for college, where she competed in national fitness competitions and won Miss Tampa Fitness, as well as doing fitness modeling for the Home Shopping Network. Then she moved back to East Tennessee, where she worked as a fitness trainer at Pilot Company Corporate Headquarters.

Jade loves all aspects of fitness, but she has a special place in her heart for the inactive. She believes fitness is for every individual. Jade was born again as a Christian in 1997 and realized her athleticism was a gift from God, and she wants to share her gift through helping others.

Jade started her company, "You Can Do Fitness," in 1997 and always wanted to write an inspirational book with daily workout videos featuring fitness for anyone desiring to be healthier. Now her new aspirations are to use social media as a platform for reaching the inactive and to work with individuals in her new gym. Jade's ultimate goal is to share with the world that *You Can Do Fitness* through inspiration, motivation, and belief in yourself.

Myriad Pro on LSI 50# Archival White
Type and Design by Karen Paul Stone

CPSIA information can be obtained
at www.ICGtesting.com
Printed in the USA
LVHW081601210223
740052LV00014B/1038